Pride and a Daily Marathon

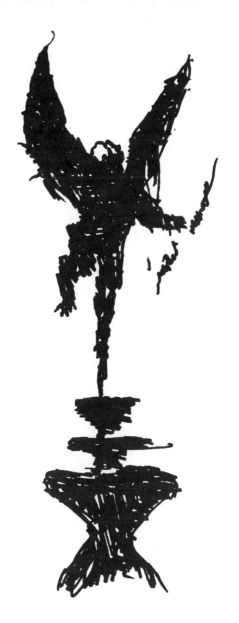

Eros. 'I drew this one evening at Odstock and it took about an hour. I was trying to find a way of employing my shaky disjointed handwriting style. It is difficult to describe the concentration required: hardly any time was spent thinking about the picture; most effort went into thinking about body position, so that I wouldn't fall over, and about gripping the pencil.'

Pride and a Daily Marathon

Jonathan Cole

Foreword by

Oliver Sacks

The MIT Press
Cambridge, Massachusetts
London, England

First MIT Press edition, 1995
First published in 1991 by Gerald Duckworth & Co. Ltd., London, England.
© 1991 Jonathan Cole

Printed and bound in the United States of America.

Library of Congress Cataloging-in-Publication Data

Cole, Jonathan O.
   Pride and a daily marathon / Jonathan Cole; foreword by Oliver Sacks.
      p.   cm.
   "A Bradford book."
   Includes bibliographical references and index.
   ISBN 0-262-53136-4 (pb)
      1. Sensory neurons—Diseases—Case studies. 2. Waterman, Ian—Health.
I. Title.
RC359.C65   1995
362.1'9687—dc20   95-13650
[B]   CIP

Contents

To Sue and Linda

For Ian

We see people buying food in the market, eating during the day, sleeping at night time, talking nonsense, marrying, growing old and then contentedly carting their dead off to the cemetery. But we don't hear or see those who suffer: the real tragedies of life are enclosed somewhere behind the scenes.

Anton Chekhov, *Gooseberries.*

There is inconsistency and something of the child's propensities still in mankind. A piece of mechanism, as a watch or dial will fix attention...; yet the organs through which he has a thousand sources of enjoyment, and which are in themselves more exquisite in design, and more curious both in contrivance and mechanisms, do not enter his thoughts. We use the limb without being conscious, or at least, without any conception of the thousand parts which must conform to a single act... by an effort of the cultivated mind we must rouse ourselves to observe things and action of which the sense has been lost through long familiarity.

Sir Charles Bell, 1833.

Foreword

by Oliver Sacks

A curious providence seems to hover over the creative encounters of patients and doctors. Did Anna O. herself invent 'the talking cure' – or was it the insight of Freud and Breuer? To what extent was Freud's thinking derived from his famous cases? Or were these cases, which to others might have seemed quite ordinary, transformed by the originality of his theories? Together Freud and Anna O. stand at the fount of psychoanalysis, just as Luria and his patient Zazetsky ('The Man with a Shattered World') produced together a classic of neuropsychology.

Ian Waterman, a patient with an extraordinary neurological syndrome, was fortunate to meet the absolutely right man in Jonathan Cole – someone who was passionately interested in neurophysiology but who, with equal passion, wished to learn the whole complexion of a life: a physician who had the detachment and skill to measure nerve conduction velocities and evoked potentials in his patient and, at the same time, the heart to travel with him and write a book which is not only a case-history but the celebration of a friend. And how lucky Jonathan Cole was to meet Ian Waterman – a man driven by his disease to a profound understanding, and a sort of heroism, who was able finally to transcend it, though there was no actual neurological recovery.

'This is a book about a person who fought with the tenacity of the damned to recover the use of his damaged brain.' So wrote Luria in his preface to *The Man with a Shattered World*. 'Though in many respects he remained as helpless as before, in the long run he won his fight.' This is true too of the hero of *Pride and a Daily Marathon*. And Dr Cole tells his story much as Luria tells Zazetsky's. Indeed his book is in the same mode as Luria's: in its combination of 'classical' and 'romantic' science, of minute neurological observation and the feel of a man's life-as-a-whole.

Ian Waterman was nineteen when he contracted his bizarre disease. A working apprentice, he had always been fit and robust. But within days, almost hours, he fell sick with a devastating inflammation of the nerves: a neuropathy which, unusually, affected only the sensory, not the motor, nerves, and especially the nerve fibres subserving touch and proprioception. He found himself deprived of feeling from the soles of his feet to his neck.

Proprioception is a vital sense which tells us the position of our limbs, informing us exactly of all their movements. It is indispensable for our motor control, for any movement we make and even for the maintenance of our posture at every second. If it is cut off even momentarily we collapse – as Ian Waterman would, if ever the lights went out. Proprioception is the inner sense by which the body is aware of itself. This is why the early-nineteenth-century physiologist Charles Bell, who was the first to describe it – or rather to infer its existence – added it to the five conventional senses. He called it the 'sixth sense', but it was a sense, he stressed, which unlike the other five, functioned automatically, unconsciously. The great physiologist Charles Sherrington (1857–1952) was the first to demonstrate its importance when he experimented by cutting sensory nerves in animals and observed the devastating effects this had on their motor control and posture. Sherrington, a fine imaginative writer, wondered how a human being would cope with such a total loss of proprioception, which had never been described. The experience, he felt, would be so remote from anything the patient had ever known before as to be 'doomed to remain indescribable'. Yet it was just this – the indescribable – that befell Ian Waterman. This book is an attempt to describe the indescribable, to articulate, through the experience of a rare and exceptional patient (and his equally exceptional doctor) a situation beyond imagining.

Few other cases have been documented of a whole-body loss of touch and proprioception – or 'proprio-blindness' (if one may be permitted to coin such a term). There have been only a few in the entire medical literature, and these contain only 'medical' details, giving no idea of what the experience is actually like – how bizarre and disabling it can be, and how difficult it is to communicate it. I saw such a patient myself some years ago and depicted her briefly in a clinical tale in *The Man Who Mistook his Wife For a Hat*, 'The Disembodied Lady'. But it was only a sketch, an intimation rather than a full analytical description. *Pride and a Daily Marathon* is the first detailed study of such a neuropathy. It is a book rich both in physiological detail and biographical narrative. Such books are rare in these perfunctory days when doctors rush in, do a few tests, make a diagnosis and rush out. They can result only from enormous labour: from thousands of hours spent with a single patient. The labour must be voluntary, a labour of love, for hospitals and research facilities can scarcely accommodate such a project in our technological age, much less support it. And yet such studies, accomplished through the selfless collaboration of rare patients and rare doctors, can provide illuminations and insights which are achievable in no other way.

A book, according to Wittgenstein, should 'consist of examples'. There are hundreds of examples in *Pride and a Daily Marathon* showing us what Ian Waterman's life is like without proprioception. At first it was scarcely a life at all. Or this was his feeling in the first months when he had lost virtually all sensory control of his body – when he could not sit, could not stand, could not feed himself, could hardly speak or swallow or control his wild movements, but flopped about, helpless as a baby. The terror of the situation is vividly conveyed: his complete bewilderment, his inability to understand or communicate what was happening to him, which made it all unbearably worse.

These first months of illness filled him with terror and perplexity. There was no recovery of sensation in his limbs and body. He had an increasing fear of lifelong disability and dependency. In these early days, when nothing could be done for him and nothing seemed to be understood, simple human kindness was all that could save him from rage and despair. But then, mysteriously, he began to get better. Or at least he began to discover new ways of doing things, now that the old 'normal' ways were no longer possible. He found he could sit up, stand up, control the movement and position of his limbs – if he watched them, if he did everything deliberately. He was learning to do anew, under conscious control, and with vision, everything that before he had done automatically, naturally and unconsciously. Thus the book is an account, not only of a loss, but of the amazing adaptations which he brought to his state: adaptations which, by the time Dr Cole met him, enabled him to go to college, to work, to drive a car, and to marry – but all this without the least neurological recovery and with an absence of proprioception as profound as before.

His adaptation is at once incredible, precarious and demanding. It is incredible, first, that he can do so much, that he is able to live, after twenty years, an outwardly normal life. My own patient Christina, in 'The Disembodied Lady', also learned to manage, after a fashion, but only while living a circumscribed and restricted life. A patient described by Purdon Martin (in *The Basal Ganglia and Posture*) was still virtually incapable of stable walking seven years after the accident in which he lost proprioception.

The precariousness is best illustrated by an example. One day in his mother's kitchen when the electricity failed and the lights went out, Ian collapsed on the floor in a nerveless heap, not realising what had happened until the lights came on again. Even sneezing, with the momentary blinking and loss of vision it entails, is a hazardous business to a man who gets no direct information from his body but has to depend exclusively on sight.

And his situation is demanding because he has to be conscious while monitoring all his activities, whereas the 'normal' way, by proprioception, is happily unconscious. He has to think constantly, and exhaustingly, how to move and where his limbs are; and if he thinks of anything else he starts to slide and fall in a heap. If he wants to talk he has to prop up his body first and stabilise it externally, so that it will stay up when he does. Every day for him, as Dr Cole says, is a 'marathon', in which he sustains himself by an effort of will – an effort which the rest of us, with our automatic proprioceptive feedback, don't have to make and cannot even imagine. What we see in Ian, in a story at once terrifying and inspiring, is a loss of the most elemental human, or animal, sensation: an almost superhuman resource and will.

At the time of his illness Ian Waterman was not a man much given to reflection, but his illness drove him to incessant questioning and self-experiment and, finally, to an understanding of himself. It made him explore his condition in a way he would never have done if he had remained in his previous unquestioning health. Such a course is described by Nietzsche, when he speaks of illness as halting the unselfconscious flow of life – its ease, its naturalness, its taking everything for granted – and as imposing on the sufferer the need to question: 'Life itself has become a problem.' Nietzsche concludes: 'I doubt that suffering makes us "better", but I know it makes us more profound.' This deepening of mind and heart is apparent in Ian Waterman. The depths were plumbed even further by his collaborative relation with Dr Cole.

Many years ago I found I was a patient myself, with a curious disorder of proprioception (due not to a neuropathy, but to a nerve and muscle injury in the leg). Luria encouraged me to write of the condition. 'You are discovering an entirely new field,' he said. 'Please publish your observations. It will do something to alter the "veterinary" approach to peripheral disorders.' Peripheral disorders, indeed, have all too often been seen as trivial and devoid of scientific, therapeutic and even human interest. *Pride and a Daily Marathon* shows us how mistaken this all is. It shows how such a peripheral disorder can have the profoundest 'central' effects on what Gerald Edelman called the 'primary consciousness' of a person: his ability to experience his body as continuous, as 'owned', as controlled, as *his*. We see that a disorder of touch and proprioception, itself unconscious, becomes, at the highest level, a 'disease of consciousness'.

Patients with such problems all too often fail to improve, and remain permanently and miserably disabled for the rest of their lives. Ian Waterman is an invigorating exception. His case shows us that, even if there is no neurological recovery, the use of vision, of intelligence, of will, can lead to a transformation and a full life. His story is an antidote to therapeutic nihilism and despair. It is a remarkable human document, showing how a human being can be thrown into a neurological hell and yet fight his way out of it to a new self-creation and life. It is, in effect, a neurological epic. Ian Waterman endures epic affliction, but he shows heroic defiance. Finally he wins, against all odds, the most obstinate of triumphs.

A brief personal note: early in 1977, Jonathan Cole, then a medical student at the Middlesex Hospital in London, came to do a neurological 'elective' with me in New York. When he came he had a remarkable knowledge of neurophysiology, having trained at Oxford with Charles Phillips, David Whitteridge and George Gordon, all eminent for their contributions in this field. But now, he said, he wanted to explore 'the other side' of neurology: how patients actually experience neurological illness, the often unimaginable worlds they are thrust into, and the equally remarkable ways they find of coping with them. It is not always easy to combine the 'two sides'. There are some physicians who have a strong scientific bent but are somewhat deficient in human 'feel' and understanding. There are others again who have this feel but are shaky in their science. It has been a delight to see in Dr Cole the steady fusion and integration of these two sides both in his work and now in a book which is at once a case-history, a physiological investigation, a detective story and a romance.

Preface

by Ian Waterman

It has been a strange feeling looking back over past events so analytically with Jonathan Cole as he researched the book. At first I was not keen on the prospect of such a searching exercise, but as time progressed I warmed to the idea. In fact I think some good has come out of it for me. First I feel that at last there is someone who really does understand the complexities of my condition. Secondly I have had to look closely at myself: not only at the physical side of how I manage my disability and the tricks I use but, more important, my motivation, strengths and weaknesses. It has done much to help me understand myself and organise my thoughts.

Hampshire, 1991   I.W.

Acknowledgements

Without the severe illness Ian suffered this book could obviously not have been written. Equally it could not have been written without his encouragement and help. To recount one's experiences for someone else to write a book about can hardly be an enjoyable experience. To do it when it necessitates remembering depressing moments one had hoped not to face again must have lead to a fair amount of rekindled distress and pain. I am grateful for all Ian's patience and humour during the reconstruction.

After reading the first draft Ian said that he had often thought he ought to try writing a book himself, but he knew he would never get round to it. He added generously that he was glad I had.

Much of the material has come from Ian's family, and I am grateful to his mother, brothers, sisters-in-law, friends and ex- wife's family for the time they gave up to talk to me and for their patience in answering questions, often about events which happened several years ago.

It is a pleasure to thank Giles Elvington, who introduced Ian and me, and Geoff Barrett for his recollections of Ian's research visit. Likewise I must thank Ian's physician at Odstock, Dr E.G. Cantrell, his physiotherapist, Miss Y. Moir, and his occupational therapist, Miss K. Fielding, for their time and willingness to remember details about Ian. If this is primarily a tale of determination in the face of a severe illness it is also the story of a triumph of rehabilitation in which these three play a large part.

I have approached Ian's illness from two complementary angles. An account of the neurophysiological loss was necessary to impart a full understanding of the effects of the neuropathy. My own interest in the subject was kindled by my supervisor and subsequent friend at Oxford, Dr George Gordon, and by Professors Charles Phillips and David Whitteridge. The book would be incomplete without thanks to them for their uncanny ability to communicate the fascination of their subject.

Of equal importance is an interest in Ian's illness from Ian's viewpoint. I have tried to approach the neurological problem, not as an academic, but humanely, as an interested friend. As a medical student I read Oliver Sacks's *Awakenings* and was deeply impressed by his understanding of what it is really like to be afflicted by neurological disease. Realising that Sacks was in a better position to explain to the patients their own illness and the snares and pitfalls the illness inflicted on them, I went to study with him on my medical elective. I learnt a great deal of neurology, psychiatry, literature, philosophy and music. But what I learnt most was to sit with patients, listen to them and to share their problems and fears. If no cure was possible, at least one could explain to them what was going on and offer to accompany them through the darkness. It was the first time I had seen a doctor shorten the distance between doctor and patient and laugh with a patient as one might laugh with a friend: a laughter which, when appropriate, did not reduce the dignity of a professional relationship but extended and replaced it with a deeper bond. I learnt much from my elective – most of all, perhaps, not to be afraid of being close to those we seek to help.

I thank Oliver Sacks also for all his comments on earlier drafts of this book and for his advice about publication. He has always been constructive and encouraging. His interest and generosity could not help but be both stimulating and inspiring. Lastly, though I was in some trepidation about asking him, since I did not wish to use or abuse a friendship, he kindly agreed to write a foreword. I am grateful to him for everything he has done for me.

Several people have read versions of the manuscript and improved it by their suggestions. I would like to thank my sister Catherine Weightman, and also George Lloyd-Roberts, Mike Sedgwick, Jaqui Porter and Patrick Scanlon. It is a pleasure to thank the several secretaries who typed various parts: Sarah Thompson, Janie Thompson, Charmian Roberts and Elaine Alexander.

After researching the book for two years, I found time to write it while on study leave in Uppsala. For his hospitality and tuition I thank Professor Karl-Eric Hagbarth. Magnus Nordin and Martin Nogues were also patient enough to listen to my ideas. The trip was made possible by the award of a Royal Society European Exchange

Programme grant and a scholarship from the Middlesex Hospital and Caius College, Cambridge.

I have been fortunate to find such an enthusiastic publisher and an editor who improved my manuscript so much while respecting its tone and character. I am very grateful to Colin Haycraft of Duckworth.

Finally my thanks to my wife Sue and daughters Eleanor, Lydia, Celia and Georgia, without whom this book might have been finished sooner – but my life would have been infinitely poorer.

Minstead, Hampshire, 1991   J.D.C.

Glossary

Ataxia: disorder of movement coordination. The word is usually applied to coordination of the body and limbs.

Axon: the long process of a nerve cell. Some sensory nerves begin in the skin of the foot and end at in the spinal cord at the level of the neck, a distance of more than a metre.

Cutaneous: pertaining to the skin.

Guillain-Barré Syndrome: an acute disease of the peripheral nervous sytem associated with an infection. It is often connected with loss of motor nerve function, so that the patient becomes weak, and less often with sensory loss. In most cases recovery occurs and is reasonably complete.

Kinetic: pertaining to movement.

Kinaesthetic: pertaining to movement sense; for example to the perception that one's leg is moving or being moved without looking.

Motorneurone: nerve cell beginning in the spinal cord and travelling out through a peripheral nerve to end on a muscle. Firing of a motorneurone leads to electrical activation of the muscle cell and hence to muscular contraction.

Neurology: that branch of medicine which relates to diseases of the nervous system. It involves both the central nervous system, comprising the brain and spinal cord, and the peripheral nervous system, comprising the nerves of the limbs and body. The diseases studied include multiple sclerosis, Parkinson's disease and epilepsy. Psychiatric illnesses like schizophrenia are excluded.

Neuropathy: disease of the peripheral nerves once they have come out from the spinal cord.

Neurophysiology: in this context the study of the functioning of the nervous system in health and illness – usually as an aid to diagnosis

– as opposed to the neurological treatment of diseases of the system.

Posture: the attitude and positioning of the body, usually considered in an upright position. The regulation of posture is normally an unconscious event.

Proprioception: perception of the position, state and movement of the body and limbs in space. Most of the information for this perception arises from muscles and joints, but in the face and hands cutaneous sensation is important.

Receptor: the specialised ending of a sensory nerve which converts a touch or stretch stimulus into a nervous impulse.

Prologue

My bleep went, again.

'There's a bloke down here who might be worth a trem,' Giles droned down the phone.

Giles was a Neurology Registrar in a busy hospital out-patient clinic, and I was a Research Registrar in Neurophysiology. I had become interested in the accuracy with which people could keep their fingers still while pressing lightly on a typewriter key. Associated with these attempts were small involuntary movements which we measured and called 'tremors' – to the cognoscenti 'trems.'

'He has a neuropathy. You might be interested.'

A neuropathy meant that damage had occurred to the peripheral nerves as they go from and to the spinal cord in the body and limbs. If the motor nerves alone had been involved, there would have been weakness; if only the sensory nerves, skin and muscular sensation (touch, pain, temperature and joint position sense) would have been affected. In most patients there is damage to both these types of nerve: the neuropathy is then described as mixed. In peripheral neuropathy the neurological lesion is usually not specific enough to allow conclusions to be made in my small experiment, and I had performed it on several patients with mixed results.

I went across to Out-patients and introduced myself to Ian. I noted that we were about the same age, 32. He was tall, wiry and slightly balding. He soon showed a sense of humour, but what struck me most was his extraordinary attentiveness to everything going on around him. After we had exchanged a few pleasantries, I explained my test and asked him if he would mind doing it. Since both the test and I appeared fairly harmless he agreed, and I showed him upstairs to the laboratory.

When I do a test I always ask the subject to tell his story in his own words, rather than take it from other doctors' notes. That way I get

1

a feeling both of the illness and of the subject's reaction to it. He told me his story briefly, and then I examined him. It was soon apparent that the damage to his nerves was extraordinarily, perhaps uniquely, specific. It had affected some of the sensory fibres, but none of the motor nerves. Fourteen years before, he told me, he had lost feeling of touch below the neck. Equally alarming was that without looking at them he had lost all awareness of where his arms, legs and body were in space.

His neuropathy and its effect on movement might be understood by physiological experiment alone. In fact his neuropathy has proved so specific that its study has allowed important insights into the normal functioning of the nervous system.[1] But the effects on him of the disease, and his attempts to come to terms with it, could not be explained simply by scientific method. Hypothesis, experiment and observation would have been inadequate for an understanding of the effect his illness had had on his life. Nor would it have explained his resourcefulness in coming to terms with it. He had suffered for over a decade and yet he had not seen a doctor trained in neurology for more than twelve years. A year before, when he became increasingly tired, his family doctor had referred him to a neurologist supposing that the neuropathy had deteriorated in the intervening decade. The neurological answer was 'No', but it was decided that he should be seen again in a year just in case.

I began asking him in detail about the illness. No less remarkable than the damage to his nerves was his long struggle to cope. The story of his rehabilitation was as important as any physiological observation we might make. The character of his illness was almost unique. Fewer than ten similar subjects have been reported in the medical literature. But it was his means of coping with the condition that was astonishing. None of the other cases was as severe, and none had been followed up.[2] Ian's loss of sensation deprived him of a vital part of normal functioning which for the most part is hidden from us. By studying his case the rest of us who are not affected may have this revealed to us. As was said by the nineteenth-century neuroanatomist Sir Charles Bell, 'we must...observe things and action of which the sense has lost through long familiarity'.[3]

I have pieced together this story by talking to Ian's doctors, physiotherapists and family, but above all by talking to Ian himself.

1

Ian the Third

Catapults and broken windows, dens and bonfires – the childhood Ian remembers is unremarkable. He enjoyed life outdoors as young boys do. He liked camp sites and houses made in the garden woodshed. He liked to use his hands. Most of all he liked to keep his rabbits, for they were alive, and his chief enjoyment was in nature.

Ian was the third of four boys, though since the fourth was much younger the elder three were closest. The three liked to cycle round the pavements of their neighbourhood in Portsmouth, often on a single tricycle making people jump out of their way. Their father had given them several warnings before they rounded a corner one day and knocked over an old lady. They knew something awful was bound to happen. After she had complained, the boys watched as their father sawed one of the wheels off their trike. Family life was never quite the same again.

Felice, Ian's mother, remembers him as we might expect, as a normal happy child. He spent hours out on his bike, cycling here and there and exploring the wood bordering their garden. He loved wildlife. This singled him out from other children in the neighbourhood and especially from his brothers. Sometimes he would be taken down to a nearby forest to see the ponies or, even better, to glimpse wild deer.

According to Felice, he fought less than his elder brothers, and then only when roused. He was not one of the usual gang, and seemed perfectly happy to be in his own company for long periods of time or to play with his rabbits. His brothers, Colin and David, remember him as a quiet boy who kept himself to himself.

Ian was always tall for his age. He played football, hockey and

3

cricket, and was a promising middle-distance runner. Such prowess is all that many boys ask for. But Ian liked sport because it was available rather than because it absorbed his interest. It was the same with friends. He had a few good friends, but he did not go out of his way to find them: he would play with them if they came round, but he was happy and content on his own.

Often sensitive children are a little lost in the hurly-burly of childhood and channel their interest into school work, but Ian was not particularly keen on academic pursuits. He enjoyed art, sport and woodwork most. His passion was reserved for the outdoors and for animals. At one stage his parents were a little worried that he was so self-absorbed and took him to their family doctor. He suggested buying him a dog to overcome his loneliness. Ian was delighted by this since he had always wanted a dog. He did not feel lonely however.

*

When he was nine, the family moved out from Portsmouth to the country. This might have seemed ideal for Ian. But he was leaving a situation he knew and friends he liked. No one really explained why they were moving. The new neighbourhood unnerved him and he wanted to go straight back. A family friend remembers him as rather moody at this time. Ian denies it:

'Twenty years ago,' he says, 'if you didn't agree with an older person's point of view, the child's comments were considered invalid and immature. It was unusual for a kid to have strong opinions, but I did.'

Ian's 'moodiness' may just have been a reaction to the change in surroundings. He soon discovered some woods near his new home and settled in to enjoy himself.

The family was not well off, and the way to independence was to take occasional jobs. First there was a paper round. Then, when he was a little older, he went strawberry-picking in the summer, often from early morning to late at night. The money was saved and put towards holidays.

He also decided to buy a dog. When anything important was bought it had to be the best. Ian decided on a pedigree English setter. His father would not hear of it and said that the garden was not fenced securely. So Ian paid for the garden to be panelled in, to a height of six feet. Then he paid for a setter from a line of Cruft's winners. He got his dog and made a point.

Ian remembers picking up Old Holborn's Cassius – 'Cas' – from the station as a pup, and from then on all his spare time was spent with him. Cas loved people, and wood – not trees, but wood: he soon destroyed the kitchen door surround, an enthusiasm which was not totally welcomed within the household.

The family had connections with Jersey and each year they would go there for a holiday. Ian by now was familiar with the countryside round his home, and he would often go for rambles and cycle rides. Everything in Jersey, however, was so much richer. There were cliffs and beaches, hills and woods, and birds on sea and land. All the family enjoyed holidays, but Ian felt an immediate love for the island. It was magical, a place of freedom and nature.

*

Gradually he thought about what he would do for a job. He had no academic inclinations, and the professions were therefore out. He had always been good with his hands and had enjoyed wood-work. His father was a toolmaker, so Ian went off to see him at his work for a while. At first he thought he might follow his father, but he was put off by the need for mathematics.

At 13 he progressed from a paper round to a job as a butcher's boy, delivering orders and helping out on Saturdays. The work was hard, but he found he loved it. There was no incongruity, he found, in loving animals and being a butcher's boy. Like most people, he couldn't slaughter livestock himself, but once the animals were dead they became to him inanimate and soulless objects.

He soon had a go at cutting up meat and making sausages. He was surprised at how much was involved in carving a side of meat into the various joints, and dressing them for the window. The precision and dexterity required were both enjoyable and satisfying. He was also good at it – the only thing, he says, he was really good at. In addition to the technical aspects of carving meat he also enjoyed meeting people in the shop. The convivial atmosphere of the butcher's shop allowed him to forget his shyness. While he was happy in his own company, he soon realised that he could also enjoy talking to customers and to his colleagues. His humour was infectious, and he was very popular.

Having found something which he enjoyed so much for itself and for the contact with people, Ian decided to become a butcher. There was no reason to prolong his schooling, and he left at 15 to become a trainee. While friends and contemporaries were still studying Ian was learning his chosen trade. He enrolled in the local college to work for a City and Guilds Certificate. He even rang up a few months before for a list of required books. He arrived at college having already learnt much of the course work, and he was soon in demand for help from fellow students. Unfortunately the course folded through lack of numbers, but he did not mind too much, since it allowed him to get on with the work itself. He had never been convinced of the importance of academic study, especially in practical subjects. Back at work full-time, he soon impressed his boss enough to be made a junior manager.

The next move was to a more senior position in a butcher's in Southampton. He used to take the first bus into town at 6.30 am and was home at about 7. He worked six days a week and rarely took his half-day off. He made some friends and would occasionally go out for a drink with them, but out of work he remained solitary. He would come home, have a meal and then walk Cas. His reading matter focused on the Meat Trade Journal and dog magazines. At weekends he sometimes had to do book-work for the shop. There was little time for dances and none for pursuing girls. His mother thinks he worked too hard for his age. But Ian was single-minded and ambitious. While others discovered new experiences, he was content to postpone serious attempts at such pleasures until he was established and successful in his job. Travel, holidays and hobbies could take second place for a few years.

*

This single-mindedness was not due solely to ambition. There were severe problems at home. All four brothers realised that as soon as they left the nest their parents would split up.

Ian's mother tried conscientiously to bring them all up, but his father never seemed sure that children were quite such a good idea. Wrapped up in his own interests, he scarcely admitted those of his children. For instance he never accompanied them to school football matches or their mother to parents' evenings. He was strict, but he never became involved in the day-to-day running of the family. On the other hand he would never let his children be put upon. He loved them, but lacked the emotional language to show it. In the Fifties he was not alone in that.

The boys knew they would have to create their own homes, and each one set off fairly early. One elder brother found a job in Jersey as a building labourer, while the youngest surprised them by announcing that he wanted to join the Foreign Legion. He did, and he has been marching happily round the deserts and atolls of the world ever since.

For Ian, being a butcher in Hampshire was all right, but he had always yearned to live in Jersey. His unsettled home situation was further reason to get away. Also, the elder brother in Jersey was returning home, so that there was less room in the house. One evening he was talking to a friend who mentioned that a butcher in Jersey was looking for an employee, with the chance of a junior partnership later. He flew over next day. He exaggerated his experience, but showed he was keen and was given a block test, in which he had an hour or so to butcher a side of meat into as many cuts and joints as possible and then dress and present them. His long hours paid off. He passed the test without any trouble and was offered the job there and then.

For years Ian's father had been pressing for Cas to be sold. Ian could avoid it no longer. The four weeks between the sale of and his leaving home he still remembers as a particularly bleak period.

*

Ian tackled his new work with his usual singlemindedness. The staff consisted of the boss, who was a master butcher, two trainees and Ian. He was working alongside the other lads, but was determined from the outset to do better than them. One of them was really a delivery man and the other was not really sure what he wanted to do. Neither minded Ian outpacing them. He was the only one who really enjoyed

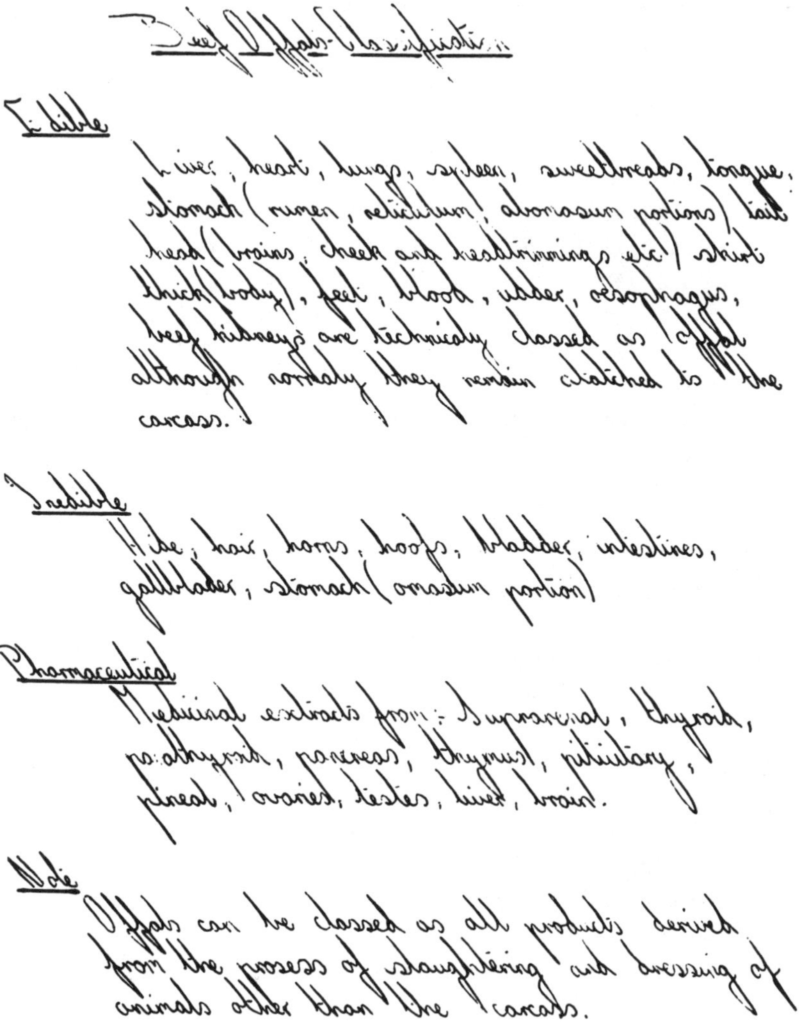

Figure 1. Ian's handwriting before the illness. This example is neater than his school work, probably because he was interested in what he was writing. The backward slant was retained after the illness and may be related to his left-handedness.

the fancy side of the work – making saddles and pineapples of lamb and crown roasts.

During the winter months the pace was manageable, but with the summer trade he was often working from 5 in the morning to 8 at night on his feet, with little time for meals. An aspect of the trade which was new to him was supplying hoteliers and caterers. He was used to cutting up twenty chops to set in the window, but now he was being asked to set up hundreds at a time. At one stage they bought a band-saw to speed things up but this was only a limited success.

With all this practice Ian soon became better and better. Occasionally he went home and compared speeds with his friends from the shop in Southampton and was amazed at how slow they were. The boss used to challenge the boys to a race to see who could cut up a piece of meat the fastest. Ian was soon the best of the boys, and then he beat his boss. After such impertinence the game was never repeated!

The long hours were not strictly necessary and the other boys did not do them. If there were ever extra duties, Ian always volunteered. Soon he felt it reasonable to ask for a bonus, which was forthcoming. The real bonus, of course, was the chance of a managership. If he did everything asked of him and more, and kept his nose clean, his boss was bound to offer it to him. Having spent his childhood holidays on this enchanted island he was back on it and determined to stay. All right, he was chained to a shop. At the end of the day he would often just wash, change, eat and sleep. Days off were often rest days. But he had found something he enjoyed and was good at.

The hours were both physically and mentally demanding. The original idea had been for the owner to pull back from the shop work and concentrate on the promotional side. He had had enough of the hours and in eight years had made enough to retire. Two friends were to run the shop as partners. However, the three did not hit it off and the friends walked out after a blazing row at a restaurant. Ian agreed with some of their grievances but decided to wait to see what happened. Without the other two the boss was well and truly stuck, as he soon realised. He promised Ian a part of the business if he would stay and man the shop. Ian agreed. By the age of nineteen he was where he had always wanted to be in a job he loved.

It seemed a trivial matter at the time that before the contract was signed he went down with flu.

2

Gastric Flu

One day in May 1971, when he was 19, Ian cut his finger. In his trade there was nothing unusual in that. Over the next day or so it became red and inflamed, and the infection spread a little way up the arm. But he continued to ignore it and eventually it disappeared. A little later – and probably there was no connection – he went down with severe diarrhoea. He felt alternately hot and cold and was very tired. Nevertheless he carried on working for a couple of days, taking care to wash his hands more often. He remembers at one stage sitting on a box at the back of the shop drinking a mug of tea and only managing to drink half of it and spilling the rest. He just thought he was being clumsy because he felt so poorly.

Eventually a workmate told him he looked really ill. Though this was the last thing he wanted to hear, he had to agree: he felt awful. He was so weak that he was not pulling his weight. Joyce, the shop receptionist, called for her doctor. He decided it was a gastric flu that was going around and advised him to take it easy, prescribing Lomotil to stop the diarrhoea.[1]

A van driver who was going into town gave Ian a lift to a chemist. After dropping him off he continued his deliveries, promising to return in fifteen minutes. Ian took his prescription in and waited outside, squatting against a wall. Overcome by tiredness, he slid down and lay in a crumpled heap on the ground. He felt stupid as people walked round him, presuming he was drunk. When the driver eventually returned, he could not get up unaided. With difficulty he was manhandled into the van before being driven back to the hotel where he was living. The two of them joked about it, but Ian's mind was working overtime; why was he losing control?

10

He was forced to take time off work. The next couple of days he stayed in his room feeling worse and worse and becoming more and more tired. The gut problems were better but the exhaustion persisted and even increased. A girl friend came to see how he was. They talked and laughed at how he would soon be up and well again. But when she left he lay on his bed in tears. He was so frightened. What was happening to him?

At one point, fed up with lying around and wondering if he really was that bad, he decided to do something. One of the odd jobs he used to do in the hotel he was staying at was to mow the lawns. Sluggishly he managed to take the motorized mower from its shed and start mowing. Slow though it was, he could not keep up with it, and he watched as it careered slowly across the lawn, fell off the edge and ended up tipped nose-down on a gravel path, like a plane that had overrun the runway. He gave up any further thoughts of work. He just managed to put the mower away and then, pausing only to admire the single swathe of cut grass in the middle of the lawn, he trudged back to his room.

He remembers looking at his watch two hours later and still feeling completely exhausted. It was a full week since he had begun to feel ill, and all he had taken was some Lomotil. The landlady came in and kindly offered to clean his room if he would get out of bed. As he went to get out he fell in a heap by the radiator like a pile of wet clothes. What was terrifying was that the reason he fell was not that he had tripped, or that he was weak or faint, but that he could not control and coordinate himself.

His landlady came back, saw Ian and immediately phoned for the doctor. The doctor gave him a full examination and sent him to hospital.

*

By the time he reached the casualty department, Ian's speech was beginning to sound a little slurred. He also noticed a tingling in his hands and feet and around his neck. This odd sensation may have come on before he reached hospital, he can't remember, but he began to think about it more then. He realised that, in addition to the tingling, he couldn't feel anything in his hands and feet. If he touched them they were completely numb. As he lay there flat on the bed, he had the frightening sensation of floating. Almost delirious from the illness, he lay there bewildered, not sure what was happening either to him in general or to his extremities in particular.

He was wheeled along corridors, up in lifts and into his ward, where he was put into bed. The screens were adjusted around the bed and he was left to get out of his clothes and into some hospital pyjamas. A nurse came back to find that he had done nothing, and began to scold him. But he had done nothing because he could do nothing. She helped him and offered him supper, which he refused, and some tea, which he accepted.

Eventually the doctor appeared, noticed his slurred speech and, much to his annoyance, repeatedly asked him if he was drunk. It took Ian some time to convince him that he was not drunk but ill. The doctor then asked if he was in contact with horses, a somewhat mystifying question. Once more there were pins and patella hammers to test reflexes. In the end the doctor couldn't tell Ian much because he hadn't seen anything like it before. He ordered some blood samples and decided to watch and wait for his seniors.

Ian remembers little else until next day. He awoke and tried to sit up, but found he couldn't. He tried to move an arm. With difficulty he succeeded, but he had no control over where it went. At this stage he remembers considering his illness with interest and some detachment, unable to comprehend its severity, let alone imagine its possible duration.

As calmly as he could, he tried to establish what had happened. He could feel nothing from the neck. Nor could he feel his mouth and tongue. Not only couldn't he feel anything to touch, he had no idea of where the various bits of his body were without looking at them. He could not feel anything with his arms, his legs or his body. That was frightening enough, but he had no awareness of their position either. It wasn't that the muscular power was affected, since he could make an arm move. But he had no ability to control the speed or direction of the movement. Any movement happened in a totally unexpected way. It was pointless to try.

He realised that that was why he had fallen out of bed. It was not that he was weak, but that he was losing the internal feedback of limb position.[2] The slurring of speech was the same. He didn't know where the parts of his mouth were and had no way of knowing when he tried to speak, or eat, whether he was on the right lines.

The consultant came and examined him again. He ordered a few more tests and was vaguely optimistic. He realised better what was wrong but he had never seen a case like it. And he had no idea about prognosis.

*

Fortunately Ian remembers little of the next few days. He can't have passed urine for some time, because the doctors were keen to catheterise him.[3] He refused, arguing that he would pass water eventually. He was frightened that, once a catheter was inserted, the bladder muscles wouldn't return to their former state through lack of use. There is no reason to suppose they wouldn't, but he was adamant. Even at this stage his obstinacy was evident. And he hated the humiliation of having it done in front of the nurses. Eventually a nurse came and ran a tap, hoping it would do the trick – it did, for she had to go off herself for a pee. Then they managed to sit him up and pressed cold hands on his lower abdomen. He started to go, and in the end filled almost two bottles. Having gone, he was not sure if he had finished. For some time after, he had strange sensations, as though he had had an accident.

They gave him a lumbar puncture, and some of the fluid surrounding the spinal cord was taken for analysis. The doctors could see what the pattern was: a severe loss of functioning of the peripheral sensory nerves. But they did not know the cause. Ian kept asking questions, but no one said much except that it was the gastric flu.

A picture somewhat similar to Ian's, except that the motor nerves are more affected, is seen in a postinfective polyneuropathy termed Guillain-Barré Syndrome, in which diagnosis is facilitated by analysis of the spinal fluid. This is why the lumbar puncture was performed. There is usually complete, or near complete, recovery.

No evidence of Guillain-Barré Syndrome was found, however. In fact the only abnormality found was that the tests for infectious mononucleosis, glandular fever, were positive. Ian cheered up a bit. At least they had discovered what was wrong. Apparently it was also known as 'the kissing disease', from the way it was thought to be transmitted. This, and the fact that there was some connection with horses, lead to many jokes about kissing old nags.

It appeared that his body's defence mechanism had produced cells which had not only reacted against the foreign glandular fever virus, but had attacked the specific nerves involved in cutaneous and muscular sensation.[4] The damage seemed to be complete, but it was not possible at this stage to say whether there might be recovery.

'The strongest memory of the polyneuritis,' he says, 'is of the total weakness and tiredness. I had been physically quite strong and active, but over the period of a week all strength and control had deteriorated. Suddenly I found myself in a hospital bed to all intents and purposes paralysed from the neck down.'

He remembers a weird feeling of his abdomen 'rippling' as he lay there. He seemed to be 'floating' on the mattress. Without sense of position or touch from his body and limbs, he appeared not to be resting on the bed. But it wasn't the relaxed floating one associates with swimming, with pleasant currents of water washing over one, but an almost unimaginable total absence of feeling. The myriad small sensations we receive from outside, or from the fleeting movements and adaptations of posture we normally make, were gone. He was in a limbless limbo,[5] an artisan of a floating world.

While he fought the awful tiredness, he had little time to consider the problem of the nerves. There were more immediate difficulties to do with feeding, washing and his toilet. The nurses had little idea what was wrong, but they knew they had to do everything for him.

*

The speech problems disappeared after a week or so, with an improvement in the facial numbness. But he still had difficulty chewing and had to be careful not to bite his tongue. He didn't know if he had chewed enough, or if the food was in the right place at the back of the mouth to be swallowed. Swallowing, once begun, seemed to take care of itself and become involuntary, but he was hesitant about everything up to that point. Food was the only pleasure left, and yet that too was denied since feeding, eating and swallowing were such chores. And he felt awkward being fed by a nurse all the time. His regular nurse would feed him while she listened to the hospital radio on earphones, heightening his feelings of isolation.

Before his illness had known some of the nurses socially. Now they came round to give him a bed bath. When it came to his private parts they would offer him a sponge, lift up the sheet and invite him to do it himself. He couldn't even move an arm for fear of lashing out uncontrollably and so had to decline, for fear of bruising himself or squashing something important. He still remembers the incongruity of having his privates washed by one of the nurses as she discussed with her friend the previous evening's episode of *Coronation Street*, or the merits of her latest boyfriend.

There was a problem for several weeks in passing urine and faeces. Neither was easy in the lying position and he had to be helped onto a commode. This needed at least two nurses. If he had been unable to move but stiff and wooden, it would have been bad enough, but he was floppy and quite unable to help by maintaining any posture. The nurses would swing his legs over the side of the bed, pick up his trunk and place his feet on the floor. Then they turned him round somehow and flopped him onto the commode.

Once a male nurse tried all this on his own, assuming that Ian could provide himself with some postural support. But he couldn't, and down he went onto the floor in a disorganised heap. He still remembers how cold the floor was. In the absence of touch his perceptions and memories had begun to be thermal. After that they would put his feet on a pillowcase on the floor, which allowed easier rotation between bed and commode. Passing urine also presented difficulties for a while, because he always felt he still wanted to go at the end. The feeling of straining was different too. But, difficult and humiliating as these problems were, they did not by now occupy his mind as much as the loss of sensation.

The nights were the worst. He would lie awake for hours. Once a young nurse came and sat by his bed, holding his hand as they chatted away. Occasionally she would disappear to see to someone else, or do a round, but she always came back. Ian remembers her as tall with dark hair and a kind face, but most of all he remembers her warm hands holding his. Contact was desperately important even though he could feel only the warmth. Her simple human kindness counted for more than all the talk and bustle he received from others.

Apart from the daily routines of feeding times, bed, bath and commode, he also had some rudimentary physiotherapy. They would do passive stretching of arms and legs, to reduce the risk of venous thrombosis and to prevent the joint contractures that often occur in immobile joints. They also rigged up a cape with slings for his arms, which could then be moved by the physiotherapist or, very tentatively, by Ian himself. He was all right while he was in the slings, but as soon as he was out of them the awful absence of feedback and the insurmountable difficulty of controlling movement became obvious again.

Talking to Ian since I have often mentioned his passivity at this time because he couldn't move, and he has always corrected me, saying that it wasn't that he had no ability to move, but that to move was useless and dangerous.

A common problem in patients without feedback is that when they are not looking at their limbs the arms and legs start to move 'on their own'. The fingers don't remain still, but writhe in small movements, and the arms may start moving uncontrollably. If he turned his gaze away for a few seconds, his arm would often come up and hit him, or someone sitting close by. This happened to several people who came to visit.

*

Ian asked his uncle and aunt not to tell his mother, but of course they did. A friend later told Ian how she had met her in the street crying. She had been walking along when she read their letter and she just turned around to go home before catching a plane. Moreover the marriage was going through a bad patch, and she decided that as a temporary arrangement she would stay with her brother on the island. She was shocked when she saw Ian:

'I walked in and saw him lying like a plant on the bed. Every nerve seemed to have gone. They even had to turn his head.'

Fortunately he never lost control of head movements, and the sister who had turned his head while he was asleep did so out of kindness, not necessity. Ian and Felice both hid their feelings and chatted about the usual things – family, the trip over, the weather. When tea arrived she had to give it to her son. That he was unable to perform a simple everyday act brought home starkly to both of them the extent of his dependence.

With the illness and subsequent inactivity he had lost a good deal of weight, and the muscles had begun to waste. It was explained to her that her son had a severe problem with the nerves, so that the messages were not reaching his brain and he could not therefore feel anything from hands and feet. Though this was true, it did not begin to explain the extent of the problem. Even though she did not really understand it all, she could see its devastating result. No idea was suggested about whether it might get better, but over the next week or so she began to steel herself to a lifetime of looking after him.

But they retained their sense of humour. On one occasion the nurses wrapped Ian in a towelling nappy (partly for decency, but partly no doubt because they didn't trust his bladder) and he was 'walked' down the ward, suspended between three nurses. His mother had to laugh, for he was like a big rubber doll, so loose and floppy it was ridiculous. With the weight loss, it made him look even more lanky and skeletal than before. But the attempt was more than a game. It was important to stand him up so that he would start readapting his circulation to the upright position, and also for his self-esteem.

Friends would visit. In fact he was often reprimanded for having too many visitors round his bed at once, as though it was his fault. On the whole he hated visitors. He didn't want to be seen like this, preferring to be ill alone. He was embarrassed by having to be fed and they all asked questions he couldn't answer. He would ask his mother to keep them away. He even suggested that she shouldn't come every day.

*

After a couple of weeks it began to seep into his mind that, though he was having treatment, there had been no significant recovery. True, he could chew better and his speech had returned to normal. But the main problem of lack of sensation from the skin below the neck and the deep tissues, muscles and joints was as absolute and profound as ever. Jersey Hospital had done all they could, but their resources were limited.

After three weeks he was transferred to the Wessex Neurological Centre in Southampton. The prospect of going to a centre which specialised in diseases of the nerves cheered him up, though the actual transfer quickly became a nightmare. The day began at 5 am. For the first time since his illness he was dressed in his own outside clothes. He was horrified by his weight loss. None of his clothes fitted at all. This was when he realised how devastating his illness was. While a hospital patient he tended to accept things as they were, but as a temporary interlude from the rest of his life. Now he was returning to normality, wearing his own clothes, and yet his condition remained the same. He was frightened – terrified.

He was wheeled out of the ward and placed in an ambulance. Rather than put him on a stretcher, they made him sit up and strapped him in round the waist. They joked about by-passing customs and smuggling booze and fags, but for Ian it was all too obviously false bravado. At the first corner, as the ambulance turned, he flopped over. Felice was with him and remembers the way he fell – just as he was, incapable of sitting upright, without any control of his own posture. He couldn't move his arm to protect himself. He fell like a baby, except that he was heavier, and more likely to hurt himself.

'I vividly remember the journey from Jersey to the Neurological Centre. Until then I had been safely cocooned in hospital, cosseted and fussed over. The journey brought home to me the extent of my problem. I can remember sitting, propped up in the corner of the ambulance. At the first bend I found myself falling over and was just saved by the ambulance man from injuring myself. I had no balance. I didn't move in time and sympathy with the vehicle. I couldn't respond and save myself from falling. I suddenly realised I had no effective control over my body. I became very confused and frightened.'

As they drove to the airport, Ian was frantically trying to control his posture inside the ambulance, while outside he could see life carrying on as normal. Then they rounded a bend, and there was the butcher's van making its daily deliveries.

In the plane things were hardly better. Though the staff were attentive, no special arrangements had been made. Again he was manhandled and strapped into a seat. He hadn't sat up like this since the illness, and without movement or control he was liable to tilt forwards at any time. Felice remembers the look of terror on his face and the icy sweat that soon drenched him. He was sick inside as they took off. It wasn't just the fear of being strapped in the plane. As the island disappeared, so everything he had wanted and worked for was left behind. For her part Felice was flying back to her husband.

At the neurological ward they assumed that Felice was the nurse and asked her to undress him and put him in a bed. The situation had to be explained, and two nurses undressed him. At least he was back in the patient role. The journey had taken about twelve hours, and he had not eaten since breakfast. Any journey is tiring, but for Ian, terrified of another fall, it was infinitely worse.

The ward was a great improvement on Jersey. There were four beds, and the nurses fussed over the patients which improved morale. They always had time to chat and made him milk-shakes whenever they could: small things, but they all contributed to his feeling that the place was well-run and that if anything could be done it would be done here.

Over the next few days he was kept busy with tests. But, as each day passed and brought with it no sign of recovery, so the likelihood of improvement diminished. The doctors at Jersey Hospital had been non-committal, but had hinted that recovery was unlikely. They were franker with his mother and told her that he would not improve. At Southampton it was the same.

When we move from one place to another the recollections and perceptions of the previous place tend to linger. So with health. We might be told in simple words that our health has altered and be able to understand this at an intellectual level, but it takes time for us to accept it – for it 'to sink in' at the deeper levels of our mind. Ian was only nineteen. A month earlier he had been fit and healthy. The hospital environment suspended his life and insulated him.

The Neurological Centre was part of a teaching hospital, training both medical students and junior doctors, and because of the unusual nature of his case Ian was much in demand. He was happy to help, especially when most of the teaching was done in small groups at his bedside. There were also grand rounds, when his case was presented in a lecture theatre. Because it took so long for him to eat and rounds usually happened at lunch-time, they would usually come to collect him midway through a meal.

Once he was taken by two doctors rather than by the usual porter and nurse. They tried all sorts of ways of transferring him from his wheel-chair to an old Morris Minor for the short trip to the theatre. He could only watch, with a mixture of amusement and terror. As they raised one bit, another flopped. In the end they abandoned the attempt and wheeled him across in his chair.

Some physiotherapy had been started in Jersey, but resources were limited. In Southampton there were physiotherapists specially trained in the treatment of neurological disorders. They had probably never seen anything like this case before, but they were better able to help than a general physiotherapist. More important, they had more time. Unfortunately many of the manoeuvres they employed to help patients regain mobility were based on the very senses Ian had lost. They did a given movement passively. That is to say, they moved the patient instead of making him move himself, so that he could learn, or relearn, how it felt and with guidance begin to do it himself. Even in healthy subjects, if the arm has not been moved for a while the central nervous system seems to need to be refreshed about the intricate details of joint angle, position and force before accurate movement begins. This update is usually instantaneous and unconscious. In Ian it was absent. All movement had to be performed with visual feedback – he had no other feedback.

The physios didn't fully understand what the problem was. Nor did Ian. But together they tried to get him moving again. They took a simple movement and repeated it over and over again, at first 'passively' but then with Ian joining in. Sometimes his effort was appropriate, sometimes not, but they persevered.

*

Between doctors' rounds, nursing, meals and physiotherapy Ian would lie in bed frustrated and impotent. He could wriggle a little, but in no positive or useful way. No one could explain why. Nights, as ever, were the worst. All he wanted was to sit up, but how? With no one to tell him, he began to plan his own campaign.

'By now I could just about organise putting something in my mouth. I would concentrate on moving the arm, bending the elbow and then the wrist, clenching my fingers tightly all the time round whatever I wanted to eat. I could just about manage it all, but as it was happening my other arm would lift off the bed by itself and float aimlessly in the air. Why the hell did it do that? All this just to enable me to eat a sweet? How could I control it? Or, more important, why should it need to be controlled? My body had looked after itself before. Why couldn't it now? What was I going to do? I could just about control my wrist moving to my mouth, bend the wrist and bend the finger. But then the other limbs would wander off, so I had to try to control them as well. I kept thinking, how the bloody hell do you do that?'

He thought about little else. He moved his legs sideways one at a time. The covers on the bed showed him where they were and acted as a hold to keep them in place. 'Next I tensed my stomach muscles in an attempt to sit up, but no luck. I didn't move. I tried again and again, but there was no real movement. The muscles started to ache. So I changed tack and tried to lift my head. I noticed that as I lifted it to check the position of my feet the top half of my torso rose from the bed. That was it, I thought: start with the head. As I tried to sit up I consciously started with the head, tucked my chin onto my chest and curled myself up. I was close to my goal but couldn't quite make it. Why? What was holding me back? My arms, my bloody arms were in the way. Their weight held me down. I checked myself over and positioned myself for another attempt. This time as I curled up I swung my arms forward. That was much better – nearly there: so close, so close. I moved my arms to a good starting position and tried again. Timing was so important. I tried again and again. Then I did it. *Did it.*'

He achieved all this with constant planning and concentration. Then once he had done it he realised he had to concentrate the same amount to keep the position. The second his mind wandered from the task all coordination was lost.

'I was sitting there swaying a bit, but sitting. I relaxed my concentration and allowed myself some congratulatory thoughts and in so doing collapsed back onto the bed.'

He still remembers the sense of achievement just in performing a useful movement after all the bewilderingly uncoordinated arm wanderings. He was also able to face the world in an upright position again. Just how he achieved it he does not know and can't explain.

'I just did it, looked at myself and did it.'

It is extremely difficult, almost impossible, to describe the mental process of selecting a given movement by activating the correct brain cells. We can't analyse consciously how we move even when the movement itself is conscious – say the turning over of a page of a book. With Ian all movement was conscious and needed visual control, but he was, as he still is, equally helpless when it comes to describing the process.

A week after sitting up in bed he managed to put his legs over the side. At the same time he was taught to feed himself, using spoons and forks with big foam handles for ease of grip. For drinking he used a baby's teacher beaker with a top and a spout. Essential aids these may have been, but he already hated them as visible symbols of his problem – he had become disabled.

The physios all had ideas about the problem, but they had little genuine insight. At one stage four of them took him to the gym. Logically they thought he would have to learn to crawl before he could walk. So they lowered him carefully down onto all fours on a mat, with cushions under his knees. But he could not see his body under him, let alone his knees and legs, and immediately panicked. He couldn't do anything in this position, and it soon made his back ache. His knees became very sore, his toes were crunched as they hit uncontrollably against the floor, and his head ached. All they had achieved was to make him more aware of his problem. The thought flew through his head: 'I am a vegetable. It's a wheelchair for life.'

He got back to the ward to find his mother waiting. He quickly concealed his fears and started to be positive about the physiotherapy. But when she went he was scared. He knew what it had taken just to sit. He could scarcely believe how severe his situation was. And he was sure no one else did either.

His mother still had a part-time job, and also a husband and two sons to look after. She visited Ian each evening and at weekends. His brother remembers, 'Mum would come home, cook us a meal and then go to visit Ian. Went on the bus, round trip of twenty miles. Don't know how she did it.'

The family would visit, and his brother was puzzled at how Ian would 'waste sweets'. They would put one in his hand and when he tried to put it in his mouth the arm would come up away from his the head and throw the sweet behind him. Meringues were crushed in his hand. They all saw it without knowing why.

*

Such trivial sideshows could not disguise the fact that no recovery in the nerves was taking place. Nor could the doctors offer any treatment – the nerves had been damaged beyond recovery.[6] That Sunday he had watched his touch and muscle senses die. The senior neurologist told him he would never walk again.

The Neurological Centre was well equipped to investigate neurological illness and to offer treatment where possible. But it could not become involved with the long-term disabled, since the beds were needed for other more acute patients who could be treated. So after five weeks Ian was discharged into the care of his mother and father. He remembers the trip home in the ambulance well. He hated it like he hated the other trips. By now there was no doubt that he was untreatable. There was no hiding it from anyone. The doctors, the nurses, the physios had all tried and failed. His discharge showed that there was little more they could do.

Felice gave up her job and they adapted the house to make the sitting-room into a bedroom. It was decorated with flowers. His mother was now his sole nurse. At 19 he had to depend on his mother to feed him, clean up after him and fetch a bottle if needed. Relatives and friends popped round and were friendly, but always there was the same question: 'What is wrong?'

If only he had known.

3

The Physiological Loss

The tingling in his arms, legs and neck and the loss of cutaneous sensation pointed clearly to a disorder of the peripheral nerves supplying the body and limbs. To understand this damage we must have a simple knowledge of the anatomy (structure) and physiology (function) of the normal nervous system.

The nervous system is conventionally divided into two: the central nervous system, comprising the brain and spinal cord, and the peripheral nervous system, the nerves which connect the body and limbs with the spinal cord. The individual nerve fibres, or axons, of the peripheral nervous system run together for most of their course in bundles which are themselves termed 'nerves'. Thus the hand is supplied by three nerves. The median, the ulnar and radial nerves each contain many hundreds of axons and each supply different areas of skin and different muscles.

In the broadest terms a peripheral nerve cell may be motor or sensory. Motor axons begin in the spinal cord before travelling via nerves to the muscles. Activation of these nerves in the cord, usually from the brain, leads in turn to electrical activation of a few muscle fibres and then to a muscle contraction. Motor nerves control not only movement and posture but also events like sweating and bladder function of which we are mostly unconscious.

Sensory nerves convey information the opposite way: from the periphery to the central nervous system. They transmit nervous impulses from specialised small receptors in the skin, in the muscles or the bladder, to give information about what's happening to and in our bodies. There are small receptors in the skin which receive touch and convert it into electrical impulses which in turn are conducted in

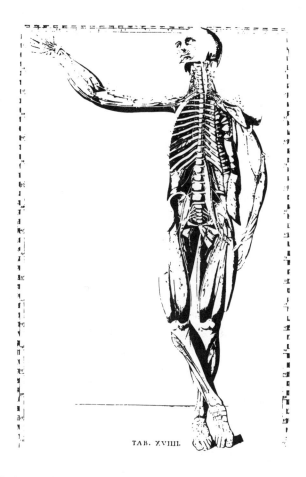

TAB. XVIII.

Figure 2. Anatomical drawing of the peripheral nervous system by Joh. Maria Lancisius, from a textbook of anatomy by Eustachii and Pope Clement IX, published in 1728. (Reproduced, by kind permission, from the collection of Dr. D. M. Balfour.)

nerves to the spinal cord and hence to the brain. Touch may be divided into light touch sensation, involving the skin, and deep touch, involving the structures below the skin, of which we are not usually aware and which seem to be less important. The touch receptors in the skin are not uniformly distributed over the body surface. They are most frequent in those areas concerned with precise movements, such as the fingers and hands, showing the importance of peripheral receptors in the control of movement.

Ian had lost all sensation of touch from below the neck because the neuropathy had destroyed those nerves transmitting that information. There are other sorts of receptor in the skin which respond, not to touch, but to pain or temperature and connect via a different class of axons to the spinal cord, but neither of these types of peripheral sensory nerve was affected.

In addition to information from the surface of the body, the peripheral nervous system also provides information from receptors in the deeper tissues: the tendons, joints and muscles. Within the muscles are small nerve endings which respond to stretch and so to active contraction or passive stretching of the muscle. There are about 20,000 of these muscle spindles, and they give information about limb position and movement. Like the cutaneous receptors they are found in those parts of the body in which feedback is most necessary. Their highest density is not in the hand, but in the muscles of the neck. Both the eyes and the balance organ in the ear require the head to be stable to function. In Ian the nerves conducting from these receptors in all his joints, tendons and muscle spindles had been destroyed except in those from the head and neck.

Muscles also contain a number of other receptors, some of which are termed 'free nerve endings' because their structure is not apparently so well-developed. Their role is less well understood than that of spindles, but they are sensitive to pain, temperature and muscle fatigue. In extreme manifestations fatigue may involve the cramp-like pain of severe effort, but it also includes the vague pleasant feeling of tiredness after a walk. These sensations are conveyed via different muscle sensory nerves to spindle information and were unaffected in Ian. As will be seen, these small muscle sensory nerves, conveying tiredness and tension in the muscles, may have become extremely important for him.

If a cross section were taken of a large nerve going to muscles and coming from skin, the individual nerve fibres would be seen not to be of the same diameter. Some would be much larger than others. The different fibres, with their different conduction velocities, are arranged in various classes, corresponding broadly to the different classes of receptor which have just been considered. The fastest fibres connect muscle spindles with the central nervous system; the slowest are concerned with pain and temperature.

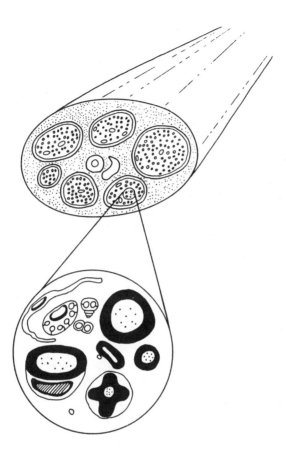

Figure 3. Diagram of a cut-section through a peripheral nerve. The whole nerve, at the top, has many individual nerve cells collected together into six fascicles surrounded by a double membrane

In the lower figure part of a fascicle is enlarged to show individual nerve fibres, in rough proportion to each other. The large nerve cells, surrounded by their myelinated sheaths (which appear in black), are shown at 2, 6 and 8 o'clock. They represent the large myelinated fibres, both sensory and motor. The small fibre at 3 o'clock peripherally represents a small myelinated fibre. The unmyelinated fibres are grouped together in the upper left quadrant.

From a rough drawing by Professor R. Weller. The figure was drawn by Mr Jack, of the Department of Teaching Media, Southampton.

On the basis of clinical testing, and from what is known of the peripheral nervous system, it may be seen that Ian's neuropathy had abolished function in all his large myelinated sensory fibres below the neck without affecting the motor fibres or the smaller sensory fibres.[1] Further detailed tests confirmed this. He did, however, have normal temperature perception, and perception of a pin prick as pain was also normal (i.e. the same on his face and on his body).

*

Now that we have seen how the various sensory receptors behave in isolation, we must ask how they contribute to perception as a whole. How do they affect behaviour and movement? Can they respond but not be perceived? Can they affect movement in an unconscious, automatic way?

Take the functions of touch. When someone taps us on the shoulder we feel it and turn round. When an insect lands on us we are aware of it and brush it off (though Ian does not). Both are examples of novel sensory stimuli which we perceive and which produce a behavioural response, a movement. Other examples are the perception of warmth and pain in the skin.

There are some sensory stimuli which if maintained are no longer perceived. Our clothes, a wrist watch, a ring, may be felt at first, but their sensations soon wear off, probably for two reasons. If the same sensory receptors are constantly activated they begin to fire less frequently: a phenomenon known as fatigue. But this is rare. As we are constantly moving, even a ring will alter its position in relation to the sensory receptors of the underlying skin. In the second mechanism the central nervous system adapts to the stimulus. The ring is not new, or interesting, and so is forgotten. Our nervous system, like our mind, is alert to change. But cutaneous sensation does not have to be felt to be perceived consciously, to have an effect on movement. Pain makes us withdraw a hand before we have time to think. Sir Charles Bell was well aware of this distinction.[2] In 1833 he wrote as follows of bed sores occurring in immobile patients who lie on the same area of skin for any length of time:

Fibre Type	Myelinated						Unmyelinated	
Conduction Velocity, m/s	120	90	60	30	6	2	2	0.5
Diameter, microns	20	15	10	5	1	2	2	0.5

Sensory
Receptor
and
[Perception]

muscle spindles
tendon receptors
[joint position sense]
[proprioception]
[muscle stretch]

cutaneous receptors
[touch]
[proprioception]

subcutaneous pressure
receptors
[deep pressure]

nociceptors
[sharp pain]

thermoreceptors
[cold]

thermoreceptors
[warmth]

nociceptors
[dull pain]

small muscle receptors
[tension]
[cramp]
[fatigue]
[effort]

Figure 4. Schematic diagram of the types and functions of the peripheral nerves. The nerves in bold type are those which Ian lost.

...the natural sensibility of the skin, without disturbing your train of thought, induces you to shift the body so as to permit the free circulation of the blood in the minute vessels: and...when this sensibility is wanting, the utmost attention of friends and the watchfulness of nurses are but a poor substitute.

Bed sores come not only from immobility but from insensitivity to the effects of being immobile. Their treatment, by regular turning, is the same today as was recommended by Bell. Ian's skin almost broke down when he was first immobile but was saved by skilful nursing.

Cutaneous sensation can lead to movement with or without conscious awareness. But what of the deep receptors, the tendon organs and muscle spindles?

There is a 'muscular sense', an awareness of where our bodies and limbs are in space in the absence of vision. Sherrington defined it as 'reactions on sense arising in motor organs and their accessories'.[3] This sense is deep within us and crucial for our normal existence, and yet we are scarcely aware of it. Perhaps Bell's greatest contribution was to describe it:

In my general course of lectures on anatomy, the great authorities made no account of the knowledge derived from the motion of our own frame. I called this consciousness of muscular exertion a sixth sense.

When a blind man stands upright, by what means is it that he maintains the erect position, or inclines in due degree towards the winds that blow upon him? It is obvious that he has a sense by which he knows the inclination of the body. It is by adjustment of the muscles that the body is firmly balanced. There is no other source of knowledge but a sense of the degree of exertion in his muscular frame.

We stand by so fine an exercise of this power, and the muscles are from habit so directed with so much precision that we do not know how we stand. But if we attempt to walk on a narrow ledge we become subject to apprehension: the actions of the muscles are magnified and demonstrative.

As Sherrington said, Bell was not the first to suppose that consciousness of the position and movement of the body is based on sensations. In *Hamlet* we have: 'Sense, sure, you have, Else you could not have motion.' But Bell was the first to postulate a muscular sense on a physiological parity with the other senses.

It becomes obvious that we must have a 'sixth sense', a 'muscular sense': so obvious that we cannot see it. This sense seems to be necessary for any controlled movement, whether of the posture or of the arms and legs. It is the function of the sensory nerves to be intimately and necessarily involved in giving information and feedback about joint position sense (proprioception) and movement to the central nervous system, so that those movements may be controlled.

More recently, paying tribute to Bell, Professor Phillips suggested that the muscular sense may be split into 'the perception of movement' and 'the perception of position'.[4] His point is that if we are often not aware of the 'muscular sense' we can hardly term it a sense at all. Better to talk in terms of what we can feel: movement and position.[5] Phillips's definitions also have the advantage of not implying that a given perception arises from a specific receptor type. It is now apparent that much of the information about finger position comes, not from muscle spindles, but from cutaneous receptors. The facial muscles have virtually no spindles; the precise movements of facial expression are under feedback control from cutaneous receptors. In contrast the larger movements which occur at the hip or elbow are likely to have peripheral feedback from spindles and tendon stretch receptors. This difference in the way feedback is organised explains why there is a large concentration of cutaneous receptors in the hand and of spindles in the neck muscles.

Recognising these perceptions does not imply that we are aware of activity in muscle spindles per se. As Phillips shows, muscles are sentient in that we feel deep pressure, cramp, fatigue and pain in them. But these sensations probably arise not in muscle spindles but in the small free nerve endings in muscles which in Ian were not affected.

Our awareness of limb position, of movements and of their speed is likely to depend on information from spindles. But before that information is presented to consciousness it is translated into a more easily comprehended form. It would be wasteful of mental effort if we had to decode consciously the barrage of activity continuously transmitted from muscle spindles into information about movement of our limbs. Unless our focus of consciousness were hugely increased, we would be overwhelmed by the amount of information.

Instead the information is built up and reaches consciousness in a complex picture. These matters were first considered by the great neurologist Henry Head:

> Every recognisable change enters consciousness already charged with
> its relation to something that has gone before, just as on a taximeter
> the distance is presented to us already transformed into shillings and
> pence.

Head gave the term 'schema' to these internal sub-conscious models
of our body position and movement, which were not thought of as
being fixed:

> By means of perpetual alterations in position we are always building
> up a postural model of ourselves which constantly changes. Every new
> posture or movement is recorded on this plastic schema, and the
> activity of the cortex brings each fresh group of sensations evoked by
> altered posture into relation to it.
> Recognition of posture and movement is obviously a conscious
> process. But the activities on which depend the existence and normal
> character of the schemata lie for ever outside consciousness; they are
> physiological processes with no direct psychical equivalent. The
> conduct and habiliments of the actor who appears before us on stage
> are the result of activities behind the scenes of which we must remain
> ignorant, as long as we are only spectators of the play.[6]

Professor Phillips talked of these 'internal brain models of our
bodies and of visual space, built up by learning during infancy and
childhood'. The schemas are not dependent only on what has gone
just before, but are a product of movement patterns developed
throughout life. By describing them as plastic Head was suggesting
that they had the capacity to alter with time. But Bell and Head made
the point that for the most part these schemas are never conscious.
The neural machinery to perform the thousands of motor tasks lie
mostly outside consciousness.

*

The damage to Ian's nerves had destroyed all feeling of touch below
the neck – this much is relatively simple to understand. But it had also
removed from him the sixth sense, the subconscious awareness of
body and joint position, the sense of movement, kinaesthesia. The
barrage of activity from the muscles, joints and skin alerting him to
changes in posture and movement stopped suddenly at the time he
went into hospital.

When we command a movement – running, say, or walking, or tying a shoe-lace – we do not have to think how to move all the muscles to make it happen. The command is split into components by our involuntary, unconscious brain. The detail of movement occurs without our conscious knowledge. Muscle spindle feedback mostly does not reach consciousness, but feeds back directly to, and only to, these subconscious programs. Without this feedback Ian found that movement was impossible to control.

We have considered touch and movement separately. Usually, however, they are inextricably linked. The main organ of touch, the hand, almost always receives tactile information associated with exploratory or manipulatory movements. Then the perception will include information both from the skin touching an object and from the receptors signalling movements. These two fuse to form a more complete tactile perception essential in guiding accurate hand movements. This fusion was termed by Sherrington 'active touch' and has been extensively investigated since.[7] The idea was clearly described by Bell, however, in 1833:

> We must not only feel the contact of the object, but must be sensible to the muscular effort which is needed to reach it or to grasp it in the fingers. Without a sense of muscular action or a consciousness of the degree of effort made, the proper sense of touch could hardly be an inlet to knowledge at all.
> The property of the hand ascertaining the distance, the size, the weight, the force, the hardness or softness, the roughness or smoothness of objects results from there being this combined perception from the sensibility of the proper organ of touch being combined with the consciousness of the motion of the arm, hand and fingers.

When we grasp a pen, or get dressed, or turn over the pages of a newspaper, or garden, we are dependent on active touch, on continuously updated sensory information from the skin and deep tissues, not only about touch, but about the relevant movements. In Ian active touch was abolished by the damage to his nerves.

We began by dividing nerves into sensory and motor branches, but the two processes, sensation and movement, are so interrelated that in functional terms the division becomes all but meaningless during normal activity.

*

The implications of this for Ian are clear. Because of his extraordinarily complete and yet specific neuropathy he had lost the ability to feel touch and to know where his limbs were in space.[8] But he had also lost the sensory input to his central nervous system to control any accurate movements,[9] whether he was sitting, walking or using his hands. Despite an apparently normal ability to produce power in his muscles he had no control over the command. He could not control the amount or extent of movement any more than he could focus the command on a single muscle. If he was asked to move his arm one way, it might go the other way, and the other arm might move as well. Even with vision to guide his movements he was helpless.

He was further handicapped by problems of communication and comprehension. These perceptions of movement and posture, and of sensation, are so intimate, so essential to us, that they seem scarcely to reach our thinking selves; and words to express them are lacking.

Though the problems are more profound than we think, we can at least imagine what it is like to be blind and perhaps deaf. Ian's loss is beyond words and almost beyond imagination. Sherrington wrote:

> Concerning this category of sensations, for their description the external world offers no adequate symbols whatsoever. There is no true basis for a convention of terms by which they may be made describable...where, in the consequence of disease, the deep organs vex the 'normal' flow of consciousness, sensations are experienced which are...singularly individual and doomed to remain indescribable.

Sherrington was a neurophysiological genius and an eloquent writer of biography and poetry. Yet he had reached that conclusion. It is scarcely surprising that a 19-year-old with little education had difficulty not only with his devastating neuropathy, but also in explaining adequately what was wrong to his family, to nurses and even, terrifyingly, to himself.

4

Down

Ian was now out of hospital: 'Here I was at home – not even in a wheelchair, as I was only safe lying down. I knew nothing constructive about my condition, only that the prognosis was grim. There was nothing the doctors could do, and they'd given up. I was on the scrap-heap. I was frightened for the future and resentful about the present. Not a happy state of mind for a homecoming.'

He didn't blame the doctors, but so much had been happening while he was in hospital that there had been little time to reflect. He had kidded himself that it was all a dream and that he would recover. Then he was discharged and able to do little more than feed himself and take a drink. As he left the ward to go home, where he had previously been well, the extent of his disability was impressed upon him.

Nevertheless it was better at first to be at home than in the ward. He was fussed over and spoilt. The food was a good deal better. He was able to watch television, which was a luxury and tolerable at least for a time.

But he soon grew bored. He was depressed and aggressive. No physical release was possible; he couldn't go for a walk or play football to work off the frustration. He couldn't even get drunk, since he couldn't hold a glass properly. He couldn't adopt either the hunched-up posture of the depressed or the strutting stance of the aggressive. He could only sit or lie there, and bellow and scream, in language both fair and foul.

'What did you do at home?'

'I used to shout at my mother. If you'd known me then I was really a different person, terrible.'

His only means of expression was verbal, and almost the only person he addressed was his mother. She had to withstand a tremendous torrent of abuse, while at the same time being Ian's only real helper. She said nothing and plodded on. Friends remember how marvellous she was. What with Ian's illness, the breakup of another son's marriage, which involved children, and her own likely divorce, she had more than enough to bear. A friend observed: 'If I'd been his mum, I'd have left home.'

But it is doubtful if anyone could just have abandoned him, with the inevitable committal to long-term hospital care. This same family friend went on to explain that, despite his illness and his painful fight with and against it, he was still recognisably Ian: 'He was a moody bugger before, and he was after. Despite the crushing illness, underneath he was just the same. Before, you'd talk to him and get sworn at, and just the same you'd get sworn at afterwards.'

'I know I was a sod,' says Ian, 'but I was also acutely aware of the pressure on my mother. I tried to hide much of the anger, fear and frustration from her, but it had to come out somewhere. It was my mum who took the brunt of it.'

Having seen her son go off to make his fortune two years before, she now saw him back home 'a cross between a rag doll and a vegetable' (equating immobility with vegetation once more). She had to wash him, shave him, put him on the commode, shower him and dress him, for he soon insisted on being dressed everyday.

The basic facts of washing and going to the loo were a huge problem and he hated the indignity of it all. Felice was amazing about that side of things. Ian was floppy and difficult to manage, but she never complained even though he only ever allowed his mother to help. The commode, which had been lent to them by the Red Cross and was kept in the corner of the lounge, was old and desperately uncomfortable, but it worked. Ian was embarrassed if people visited when it was still in the room, and it was worse if visitors arrived just after it had been used. He remembers the disappointment if he couldn't perform in the evening before going to bed, knowing that he would have to go during the next day, with the lingering, faecal smell. He developed a strong bladder for a similar reason.

Felice would pick him up so that he was in a vertical position and try to make him grip her round the neck or body. But though he could grip, he had no idea how much force he was producing. His only feedback was when she choked for breath or gasped with pain. Somehow they managed. She used to pray and pray every day: 'Let him be better. Please, a miracle.'

'My worst thing,' she said, 'was getting him to the loo. I used to pray, 'Let him just be able to do that.'

Hair washing was difficult too, because he couldn't bear to have shampoo or water near his eyes (or he would have to shut them and lose his only remaining clue of where he was).

One day soon after arriving home, he fell between his bed and the wall. He ended up wedged, unable to move or even to understand his position. He was terrified. Thoughts of what an odd place to die filled his mind. Felice couldn't get him out and had to ask for help from the neighbours before he was freed. Even home – even bed – had its dangers.

Unable to move, Ian spent his first weeks at home propped up watching television – or just propped up, allowing his thoughts to be focused on himself, to fester and to increase his bitterness and anger.

When Felice had gone out to Jersey to see Ian soon after the illness she had taken many of her things with her. It was to have been the separation before a divorce. When he showed no sign of recovery the plan had to be changed. His father had not only his wife back but Ian as well, whose major contribution was to make the living room untidy. All things considered, there was a big incentive for Ian to improve so that he could leave all this behind for the second time.

*

Work had enabled him to meet people, so escaping from his shyness, and to move to Jersey. Now the illness had deprived him of his job, his independence and his ability to move. All it had given him was time and solitude. It had driven him back to his childhood and adolescent loneliness.

His problem was made worse because, apart from his looking thin and tired, there was no visible sign of the illness. It remained insuperably difficult to explain:

'How are you?'

'I don't know.'

'What's the matter?'

'I'm not sure.'

He would say that the nerve ends had gone in his fingers and toes. He was exploring the consequences of the loss of proprioception almost without knowing it, but it was a sense so basic and yet so difficult to explain that he found it impossible to communicate. He often gave up, increasing the distance between himself and others and worsening his depression. His brothers occasionally took him out for a drive, but otherwise he stayed at home. For weeks on end he saw only his family, except for his visits to physiotherapy. Friends tried to call round and see him, but he discouraged it, not wanting to be seen in this condition.

Family life wasn't a haven either, nor was it comfortable. All the time he was at home he felt guilty:

'An awful thing to feel so damned guilty about the situation all the time. Very negative. You end up sort of paranoid, I suppose, but that's how it was. You feel such a burden. Disability never affects just one person, it has its repercussions on all those who come into contact with it. I ended up feeling that all family arguments were directly due to me, which was crazy because we had always argued.'

He became terribly depressed, but always tried to keep it inside him. He felt guilty about all the problems his disability was causing in the family. It was because of him that his mother had had to return to his father. He would cry at night when everyone was asleep. 'I was better that way. Guilt is often a stalking horse for paranoia.' He began to doubt that his parents were being honest with him: 'I felt that secrets were being kept from me about my disability, but of course they weren't. I would quiz my mother if she spoke to the doctors or anyone about me, but as usual no one had said anything. At first I used to think the illness might be terminal, and that this was being kept from me out of kindness. My mother must have been driven mad. I always expected her to tell me everything, which she did, but I never really opened up to her. I was doing to her exactly what I thought the medical establishment was doing to me, and of course it was a vicious circle. Mad, when you look back on it.'

Felice could see something of what was happening but wasn't always able to reassure him because he never managed to open up and talk about his feelings. He wished he could talk more, but he was stuck between the need to express his worst thoughts and his fear that bringing too much out into the open would somehow make those thoughts a reality. Instead he worked at keeping the outward appearance of happiness and optimism, thinking it would be easier on those around him.

People would ask Felice what was wrong, and she would be stuck too. She knew he had lost feeling and coordination, but more than that was difficult to explain. Seventeen years later relatives and friends were still quite unaware of the extent of the problem, saying that they had never really understood.

A family friend came round several times to invite Ian to her wedding. He refused: he would not let people to see him in this state and it would also have meant using the despised wheelchair, which he rarely did. He would not use it around the house. He even made the ambulance men carry him rather than use it when he visited the hospital. Some time later he did go to a wedding, but he just sat there, saying little and moving not at all.

Often it was all too much for him and he would break down and cry. Trying to comfort him as best she could, Felice would be told to bugger off. She did her best, ignored the abuse and went round to friends before letting her own tears fall.

When she gave up her job she soon found money short. So they applied for help from Social Security. The GP wrote to a panel of experts who considered the case. Ian was not then a registered disabled person. A man came round to assess him and, not surprisingly, was quite incapable of grasping the problem. Ian was judged not to require a nurse twenty-four hours a day – which was just as well, since Felice needed some time off – so he did not qualify for a Constant Care Allowance. Anyway, as they pointed out, they had not had such a case before and so there was no precedent.

They laugh about it now and laugh about the poor man who had no idea of what Ian's illness was. But at the time the failure to secure extra cash was a severe blow.

Though discharged from hospital as an in-patient, Ian was still being followed up in the out-patients department. In hospital he would allow himself to be placed in a wheelchair, and he was wheeled in by Felice to see the consultant. One morning, after a short interview to discuss his 'progress', the doctor asked him to do a few simple arm movements, and then to do them with his eyes shut. Both he and Ian knew the futility of it. So at first Ian was puzzled at the charade. But as he made his attempt at movement with eyes shut, he heard whispers and knew it was a signal for his mother to stay behind at the end.

Sure enough it was the sister who wheeled Ian out while Felice stayed behind. He sat there thinking: 'Well, he'll be telling the old sausage the worst now.'

After five minutes Felice came out in tears. Neither spoke, and they went home in silence. The doctor had given them both his expert opinion in good faith and for the best of reasons: to prepare them for the inevitable. Ian was not sure he believed it. He *may* have believed it, but he refused to accept that he believed it - he could not afford to. He was worried but he would not show it to his mother. Likewise right from the start she had a vision of herself tending a wheelchair-bound son for the rest of her life. She had never mentioned that to him, and was not going to now.

It isn't unusual in medicine for the now famous 'conspiracies of silence' to evolve when someone is faced with the unbearable, a fatal illness or an insurmountable handicap. But it isn't always wrong to avoid a frank discussion. In this case, by not talking they never admitted to each other that what the doctor had said was true. By reaching no conclusion about the future, they allowed the possibility of altering it. Their silence was a conspiracy, if not of hope, at least of defiance – of hope suspended.

'We had a mutual unspoken agreement, I suppose. I firmly believed that my determination to regain independence would have been reduced had I accepted my circumstances and felt more comfortable about the whole situation. As it was, I was determined not to be a burden. This drove me forward.'

*

Week followed week. Month followed month. Ian remained practically immobile, dependent on his mother for movement, and imprisoned in the house. Convicts are sent to jail, are 'given time'. This means that they serve the sentence locked away, unable to involve themselves in the usual business of life. Such time is irreplaceably taken from them. But by being locked up, often for twenty to twenty-three hours a day, they are also 'given time'. In a small cell with nothing to do boredom is inevitable, and unoccupied time passes slowly. With most useful occupations removed, prisoners 'serve time' in the sense of being at the mercy of it.

For the prisoner, the cause of his incarceration is clear, and an end may be in sight. But Ian was denied involvement in life and given time to think and ruminate upon the illness, its duration stretching out indefinitely. This gnawed away at him hour by hour, day by day, ceaselessly. The anger, the frustration and the self-pity threatened to destroy his dignity, his self-esteem and, finally, himself. The only direction he could turn was in on himself, and this merely made things worse.

Television could not divert his attention for long. He tried reading, turning the page by licking his fingers. He kept dropping the book and could never find the right page again, so he read the same bits over and over. At least it demanded more active involvement than the screen. He chose prisoner-of-war novels, for obvious reasons. Lastly there were the huge jigsaw puzzles. A friend remembers the hours Ian would sit doing these puzzles. From the start he chose tasks which were difficult but required him to use his hands. The puzzles kept his mind occupied as he struggled to work out how to pick up the pieces. 'I could see the piece I wanted but it was difficult to get it. Even now it's difficult. I used to wet the end of my finger and aim it at the piece I wanted.' He would take weeks to complete a puzzle and refused help.

*

He hardly ever went out. 'No. I refused flatly. At that stage I found my disability hard to accept. I thought, "I'm a cabbage now, they don't expect me to walk again." [Again equating being a vegetable with absence of movement: I move therefore I am; I don't move, therefore I am not.] I was frightened. In hospital the thought remained that the illness would end, but at home that hope had vanished.'

As an attempt at bathetical humour, I remarked that it must have been worse than acne. He replied that after the illness he had severe acne as well!

A trainee social worker used to come round to visit, chat and offer help. He would talk for hours about the condition. Every time he came he would ask the same questions, and his lack of interest was soon apparent. Ian just remembered his prodigious appetite for tea and chocolate biscuits. He asked him once for a ramp for the front door, but it never arrived. He was also annoyed that he insisted on doing bits of the jigsaw puzzles to help out. If Ian saw him coming he would tell Felice to say he was asleep. At one stage the man decided to get Ian to touch-type. He even brought round an old typewriter. When Ian said touch-typing was out he asked why. Ian explained, and he said, 'Oh really, I didn't realise that.' Ian exploded: 'What the hell were you doing on all the other visits when we've discussed the problem?'

The man didn't come back.

*

By Christmas Ian had been at home for about four months. The sight of all the decorations just increased his sense of loss – his loss of sense. He thought quite seriously of ending it all, but knew he would never be able to reach any bottles of tablets, or be able to unscrew the bottle tops. But he could get drunk. As it was Christmas, there was some alcohol in the drinks cabinet, and one night when his parents were asleep in bed upstairs he slithered out of bed and across the floor to try his luck. He managed to open the cabinet and just lay there, drinking whatever there was. Felice remembers:

'About 3 am we woke up, disturbed by a noise. My husband went downstairs and came back saying, 'Your son is drunk.' Well, he was *his* son as well, but I had to do everything. I don't know how he'd managed to unscrew the bottle tops, but there were empty bottles everywhere. (He hadn't – he'd only taken corked bottles, and he soon felt sick, so he tried to find something to vomit into.) I came downstairs and he was lying there with his head stuck in a wastepaper basket completely unable to move. I had to get his head out, and somehow get him to bed. He was so like rubber. All the work we'd put in to try and improve him – everything had gone. It was like being back at square one.'

Once sober, Ian was terrified. It was six months since the illness, and he had learnt to sit, to feed himself, and to slither rudimentarily. All these skills vanished for days after the alcohol. He had learnt how fragile his memory and re-acquisition of movements were. It was frightening to be shown that whatever skill he had learnt could be lost so easily.[1] From then on all drink was kept upstairs. He realised that another release, albeit a temporary one, was unavailable.

Though totally reliant on his mother, Ian insisted on maintaining what independence he could, to the frustration and exasperation of those around him. He hated signs of disability and did all he could to disguise them. After a few days at home he had refused the padded cutlery. He had many accidents, and many cold dinners, but eventually mastered the use of an ordinary knife and fork:

'We had hundreds of arguments. I preferred feeding myself a cold dinner to being fed a hot one. This insistence on doing everything I could for myself caused problems for my mother, and we argued often. But I knew I had to try and regain some independence.'

Similarly he hated the baby beaker, and after a few days insisted on an ordinary mug. He spilt dozens and dozens of mugs of tea down his lap. He soon decided to let the drinks cool first.

He always insisted on being dressed every day. Soon he wanted to dress himself, which caused problems. The downstairs lounge could not be used by anyone else while this was going on and it was a slow and laborious task. He would rarely accept help – and rarely accept defeat. It might take twenty minutes to put on a sock, but he would do it. He would sit on the edge of the bed to dress. One morning Felice was in a hurry but Ian still insisted on doing things for himself. Disaster inevitably occurred. He managed to get the jumper stuck on his head. Tugging and wriggling, and becoming angrier and angrier, he fell off the bed. This sort of thing was fairly common: it just meant loss of pride. But this time as he went down he knocked over the tea, the toast and the bedside table. And as he was on the floor Felice had to lift him back. There was bad temper all round. She thought him stubborn: he wanted her to accept his need for independence. As in most family arguments, both no doubt were right.

With help he taught himself to 'bum' around the house, and soon set off into the garden. He refused to allow a ramp or bars to be constructed to help him around. There were many arguments. His mother called him bloody-minded and arrogant. What others thought can only be imagined. Still only 19, he was hanging on as best he could:

'I was painfully self-conscious about my disability. Even when I had learnt to overcome a problem I wouldn't show how clever I was and perform the trick in public. I was struggling for normality, and a show like that would confirm the very disability I was seeking to deny. One of the things that kept me going was my pride, my bloody pride.'

*

Felice realises now that he was right. It would have been easy to accept the help, accept the wheelchair, and get on with the new life of disability. After a period of anger and grief he could have sat in the chair and faced the world as a disabled person. But he refused to embrace less of a life than he had known before. He did not know what lay ahead, or whether any recovery was possible, but until he did he was going to be defiant. Depressed he was, but he was never beaten.

One day he hit on the idea of scattering blankets from the bed onto the sitting-room floor to make a soft path and practise taking steps Douglas Bader-style. When everyone else was in bed he folded his blanket on the floor and marched up and down on his knees. He was wobbly, exhausted and alone; but it was Christmas Eve – the stomping was a present to himself. He promised himself that next year he would be standing. He spent hours walking on his knees to get used to it, mostly at night. He never told anyone what he was doing. His thoughts of recovery he kept to himself: to avoid fuss and to avoid failure.

One ally was his GP. Janet Shakespeare, a woman of formidable spirit, had just returned to Britain after eighteen years in South Africa. It was to her that Felice turned in her moments of despair. She received, not pills, but sympathy, understanding and, most precious of all, time. When cure is impossible, the least a doctor ought to be is an informed and helpful confidante and friend. Dr Shakespeare often called to see Ian on her rounds. If he was still in bed she would make him get him out. If he wasn't dressed she would make sure he was. She encouraged him constantly and told him he would walk again. (Perhaps it was just as well she was no expert in neurology, or she might have known better.)

At a crucial time, when Ian was having to defy his illness almost single-handed, she gave him support and hope. Best of all, she had time to listen.

Slowly, almost imperceptibly, Ian's mood changed. He was capable of only so much grieving, mourning and shouting. He began to realise that the anger was consuming him. What he had begun as righteous rage against a personal injustice had rotted and become destructive:

'Being bitter doesn't work. If you want you can get all the sympathy in the world. But it's not productive.'

This did not lead him to accept his disability. The defiance remained, and so did much of the bitterness.[2] But he began the long process of gaining perspective and analysing his condition. He had seen what six months of railing against his illness had done to him, and to those around him, and he did not like it.

On one of his many visits to the hospital in the ambulance they stopped at a local geriatric ward to collect a patient and his escort. The escort turned out to be a girl whom Ian had been to school with. She did not recognise him at first, and he was in two minds whether to speak to her from his stretcher. But they started talking and she promised to visit him. Some time later she turned up unexpectedly, and they had a good chat about old times. Suddenly it hit Ian that, while everyone else was getting on with their lives, he was just vegetating. The girl saw he was upset, and he told her about his frustrations and how isolated he felt because the doctors seemed unable to tell him anything constructive about his illness. She replied that, if they were unable to tell him anything positive, why believe the prognosis was so negative? She didn't come again, but Ian often reflected on their conversation. The logic may have been tortuous and her understanding of the neurology vacuous, but maybe, just maybe, she was right.

Felice remembers an old family friend coming to see him one day. Quietly and gently he put a pencil in Ian's hand and guided it through a letter or two. Ian was incapable on his own, yet with help it was not as impossible for him to write as his mother had imagined. This was the first time she realised that some useful recovery might be possible. This man, in five minutes and with scarcely a word, had shown her that her son's defiant hope might not have been in vain.

At about this time Ian decided to keep canaries. He says in retrospect that it gave him a reason to get up in the morning. He was beginning to think beyond his illness. With Felice's help he designed a cage, and his father built it while Ian directed, propped up against a wall. Friction soon developed, since Ian knew exactly what he wanted and would not allow his father to cut corners. But eventually the cage was completed. Ian had many happy hours inspecting the birds. Attempts at breeding were unsuccessful, however, due to what Ian thinks was the only homosexual canary in Hampshire.

Felice helped with movement exercises which Ian had devised. She was often bruised as she was kicked off the bed. Throughout this period Ian went faithfully to physiotherapy. There the approach was to perform simple patterns of movement and to repeat them endlessly.

'They would move a leg in a certain way and repeat the movement time and time again. I'd try to build up a pattern in my mind, and of course try to build up the muscle itself. I'd lie on a bench and they would grab an arm and I would push against them as they pulled and then pull against them as they pushed. I couldn't say at the time that I felt I was getting much from it, but looking at how things have gone it was one of the better approaches.'

Passive movements were useless, everything had to involve him in effort.

'Yes, I had to push or pull, so I did get some feedback from the tiredness. Thinking about it, that's perhaps how it went. They used to lay me on my back on the floor and put my knees up with my feet still on the floor. I'd close my eyes, and my knees would fall over. We'd see how long I could do it for, and see if there was any improvement in control without visual feedback.'

'How did you stop them floating away?'

'I never did.'

'How long before the physios gave up?'

'They never did, but we moved on to other things. Repeating movements was OK if I put effort into it. Sometimes they'd move my arm in and out with little effort. I had to try and put effort in to gain any advantage.'

'There were some gorgeous girls. They used to pull my arms away from me and say, 'Resist me, resist me.' Well, underneath the neuropathy I was a normal, rampant 19-year-old. I just said it was too difficult to resist.'

The ambulance drivers were good fun with Ian and over the months they built up quite a relationship. Ever ready for a joke, they once brought him back fitted up with inflatable splints on arms and legs. They called Felice out to the ambulance and gave her some story about there being a problem at the physio. When she saw Ian, the look on her face was superb. She was completely taken in. Everyone laughed about it for ages.

The physios who treated him as an outpatient were marvellous. They went over the same routines again and again and encouraged him constantly. They were also young and attractive. It was a great break from the routine of home.

*

One day he saw his father sitting in the reception area. He was astounded since no one had mentioned he would be there. According to the physio he was just checking to see how his son was progressing. Ian managed to do some routines but was so angry and embarrassed by it all that he did not perform very efficiently. He hated anyone he knew seeing him practise. His father had meant well, but it had all been done rather crudely. The physio ushered him out and the session continued. At the end Ian talked for a long time about why his father's presence had so upset him and about the situation at home.

The physios and doctors in the rehabilitation department saw how profound his problem was. They could see that three hours of their time a week was not enough. They had now learnt of his poor home situation and were impressed by his determination. The obvious thing to do was to send him on a course of in-patient physiotherapy.

Dr Graveson, his consultant, agreed, and a letter was written to the Regional Rehabilitation Centre:

'This lad is just about the worst case of polyneuritis we have ever seen. It damaged his sensory fibres. He never had any motor weakness, but total loss of joint sense. He has not recovered very much. I do not think he is going to get much better, but he is a nice lad and I hope you will be able to do something for him.'

Ian puts it more bluntly:

'They saw they were getting nowhere, and they also saw the problems at home, so they arranged for me to leave.'

They and Ian were fortunate in having a hospital devoted to rehabilitation twenty miles away in Hampshire. Ian went there having sworn his way through seven months of hell at home. His mood was lighter than it had been at Christmas, and the worst of the depression had burnt itself out. He was ready for something new, though he remained sceptical that anything would come of it. The doctors, whom he had been brought up to consider the epitome of knowledge, had not been very helpful before. What could a new set do? The alternative, though – of staying where he was – was too awful to contemplate.

5

Outward Bound

The village of Odstock lies near Salisbury, about twenty miles west of Southampton. It is sandwiched between steep downland and a small trout river, which by bursting its banks each winter has protected itself from development. Its priorities are clear. At one end is the church, at the other a beautiful Glebe House, and in the middle, at the crossroads, stands a pub.

Odstock is separated from the city by a hill, on top of which a services hospital was built during the war. Since then Odstock Hospital has gradually been enlarged, and has been used for various specialties of medicine. It contains a famous Plastic Surgery Unit, a Spinal Treatment Centre and the Wessex Regional Rehabilitation Centre. Because it has a fair amount of land it is now being expanded into Salisbury's main hospital. When Ian went there, however, it still consisted almost entirely of single-storey wartime huts.

The regular ambulance crews who had taken Ian to physiotherapy took him to the hospital. Thinking it would be a more pleasant run, they drove through the New Forest. When he arrived he was less than impressed, since he was assigned to an old army nissen hut. It was 20 March 1972 and he had been at home with his family, refusing to see almost everyone, for seven months. It was more than nine months since the start of his illness.

He soon cheered up. The staff were trained to be concerned, not with acute disease and its diagnosis and immediate treatment, but with the longer-term effects of disability. This made them more relaxed and approachable than staff at the other hospitals.

Ted Cantrell was the doctor who admitted him. In his notes he described Ian as a pleasant young man with a strong will to get on.

For Ian's part he was delighted, at last, to meet a doctor with a sense of humour. Dr Cantrell asked if him if he had shaved that morning. He had, but as always, not very well. 'Don't worry,' said the doctor, as he stroked his full beard. 'You made a better job of it than me.'

The notes describe his reflexes (all absent), his loss of skin sensation and proprioception and the fact that he was ataxic. He could transfer from bed to chair and dress himself (and that took twenty minutes). He could feed himself and drink from a cup. He could type but not write. He was 'still too ataxic for safe wheelchair manipulation'. In fact he could sit in a chair but could not propel it with his hands at all. Finally, 'he has been very bored at home'. The aim was to get him occupied both in physiotherapy and in rehabilitation, the former to build up muscles and help him regain movement, the latter to develop skills such as writing.

Yvonne Moir, the chief physiotherapist, obviously belonged to the forceful-but-kind school of physiotherapy. She inspired a deep loyalty among colleagues and patients alike. She remembers him well:

'Dr Graveson was pessimistic about his future. But we never turned anyone away. He was young and had no chance of returning to his trade. Our aim was to try to get him back to some sort of employment. Even if he could never live independently, he needed to earn a living.'

Ted Cantrell remembers two problems that come up again and again in rehabilitation – the disability and the person's response to it.

'I hadn't seen anything like it, and didn't realise at first how crippling the loss of sensation was. He had no balance, no control at all.' (When I talked to Dr Cantrell many years later he had forgotten that the problem was in cutaneous touch as well as proprioception.)

'In character he showed two levels. Superficially he was jokey and slightly extrovert. But very soon you saw that there was a profound unhappiness underneath. His family was broken and disrupted, so that despite his gallant mother he was more on his own than he might have been. He was also extremely depressed and couldn't see what to live for. He had left school early because he couldn't stand it, and now the only job he had wanted was closed to him.'

When asked what he thought might happen to Ian, Cantrell said that he would improve to the extent of being able to do a limited desk job, but in a wheelchair. Yvonne Moir agreed. Later they both had to be pressed to admit that that had been their opinion. At the time their professional judgment was necessarily open-ended and based week-by-week on whatever progress was made. They did not, and do not, set an absolute level of achievement for their patients. They see how far each patient can manage to go by coaxing and encouragement.

As he needed full-time nursing to help him dress, wash and go to the loo, Ian was placed on a general medical ward. Next to his bed they put a wheelchair, and there it stayed. If he had to go down the ward he would always try to get them to wheel him on the bed rather than use the chair. Likewise he tried to use the commode near his bed with the curtains round rather than be wheeled to the loo.

Every day he was taken across for therapy. At first physiotherapy dominated. He would be placed on a chair and made continually to extend arms and legs. Laid on his side, he had to push out sideways against someone in a crab-like movement. He was encouraged to bum his way round the gym.

*

He had been seven months alone at home. Now he had a whole team encouraging and helping him. The physios did not really understand what was wrong, but they regarded him as a Guillain-Barré patient – someone in whom neurological improvement was the rule and in whom functional recovery was expected. He was forced to be occupied all day and made to join groups of other patients. He was attended by young enthusiastic physios.

The re-emergence of even simple movements was a difficult matter, given the prolonged immobility and loss of internal feedback. In normal subjects if the arm hasn't moved for a while the nervous system needs, as it were, to be 'refreshed' about all the intricate details of joint angle and position before accurate movement can begin. This update is almost instantaneous, but in patients with neurological disease, for example stroke victims, when a side of the body is paralysed or weak, this is not the case. The eminent Norwegian neuroanatomist Alf Brodal suffered a stroke with profound weakness and apparently normal sensation. He wrote an eloquent paper on his recovery. The value of passive movement in physiotherapy has been debated, but Brodal was in little doubt:

At the beginning it often happened that the patient, even with his strongest effort, was unable to make a voluntary movement of a particular joint, but when the movement had been made passively a couple of times, the patient was able to perform the movement, although with reduced force. Subjectively it was clearly felt as if the sensory information produced by the passive movement helped the patient to 'direct' the 'force of innervation' through the proper channels. It may well be that there are subtle neurophysiological mechanisms in this 'facilitation' of movements. From introspection it appears, however, that the subjective information about the movement to be executed, its range and goal, is an essential factor. The phenomenon is probably parallel to the learning of all motor skills.[1]

The paramount importance of feedback from the limb in the process of relearning is stressed. In 1854 an eminent physiologist, George, had said: 'Only when we move a limb do we become conscious of its existence.'[2]

For Ian, this feedback had vanished as those senses died that Sunday afternoon. Passive movement would be of little use. Physiotherapists could help him, but only to help himself, since all movements had to be made actively under visual guidance. What he got out depended absolutely on the effort he put in.

Brodal went on:

Among an original multitude of more or less haphazard movements, the correct ones are recognised as such by means of the sensory information they feed back, and this information is later used in selecting the correct movements in further training.

Ian had been denied this selection process. Perhaps it was just as well that neither he nor the physios had read Brodal, so they just got on as best they could. There were no words to explain to them what to do: they just took a movement and repeated it time after time. Ian was being encouraged to do much more than he had done since the illness. Some ideas were of little use, and then he would suggest something else. Progress was slow, very slow, but at least it was progress.

Within days they had dragged him out of his chair and stood him up, albeit at wall-bars and with people holding on. Within two to three weeks he was able to get up on the bars himself, though only slowly. At first four of them helped him, but then there were only two. The floors were wooden and splintered. When he asked why, Yvonne

Moir replied, 'To discourage patients from falling.' Ian thought this was a joke, but he was not certain. They used to get him standing and holding onto wall-bars, and leave him there, with a wheelchair behind in case he fell. He can remember the bars inches from his face as he watched the sway, trying to learn how to stand.

At other times they would lie him on his back and get him to move arms and legs to command. Sometimes he would work with just one physio on the mats while he moved arms and legs on command as she applied resistance and pressure. It always seemed to end up with her squatting or standing just above his head, and he would be mesmerised by her turquoise silk underwear. He remembers his disappointment the day the uniforms changed and everyone turned up in dark-blue trousers. They would make him kneel and after a while try to catch a ball or a bean-bag. Their aim was to teach him to move more freely. But for Ian the point of the exercise was very different. He was learning to freeze movements and concentrate on more than one thing at a time. Often the physios did an exercise for their reason, while Ian did it for another. They progressed in parallel. The important thing for Ian was the encouragement he received. There was a set of steps only six-up, six-down which they encouraged him to ascend. There were arm rails but the steps were open. Ian was terrified but had a go. By the time he left he had mastered them, but they always terrified him.

*

While all this activity was going on in the gym Ted Cantrell and the nurses were busy planning Ian's living arrangements. After two weeks he was moved from the acute medical ward into a hostel for long-stay patients, sharing with people with badly broken legs, hand injuries or strokes. During the day they had a full routine of physiotherapy – daily living activities, workshop and crafts – but at night they were left alone.

The reasons for moving him so soon were not that the ward was inappropriate and the bed needed for others. They had decided that Ian was a loner and they wanted to throw him into social contact with his fellows. As they saw it, the other patients would keep a proper eye on him. They allowed him to have a go at things but would not let him try for too long if it was obviously hopeless.

While some of the exercises were good for him, some were pointless, based on a misunderstanding of the problem.[3] But what they brought was a welcome enthusiasm and an expectation of improvement. This contrasted with the attitude at the Neurological Centre where the doctors were pessimistic. Expectation of failure usually inhibits.

During the first week they tried to improve his sensation with a vibrator on the skin, with rubber spikes to develop feedback. But of course he felt nothing. They tried him crawling on hands and knees. Again this was unsuccessful since it was not a favoured posture with Ian. They focused on touch by giving him various shapes to feel with his eyes shut. He soon learnt to distinguish circles from cubes and stars because they were made of different material; and wood made a different sound from cardboard when touched and rattled. This progress encouraged them to believe that some recovery was taking place, until he showed them how he had done it.

*

For all their help and ideas Ian began to realise that the physios had no real understanding of what the effect of the neuropathy had been. He worked out that the best way to proceed was to do everything he was asked to do, but to use it for his own purposes rather than the ones his teachers imagined it was for. They thought he was improving because the neuropathy was improving, and that he was developing some feedback. He knew there was no recovery, and that if he was improving it was because he was learning to use what he had left to more effect. This crucial distinction he kept from them, because he found it so hard to express. It did not matter much either. They were so enthusiastic and kind that it created the ideal safe place for him to experiment.

Occasionally his progress clashed with his teachers' view of it. They didn't realise how tired he became with all this extra movement and hence extra thought. Doing something the first time required only a little more mental effort than doing it on subsequent occasions. He took short rests when he could, though he knew that the physios thought he was slacking. It was yet another aspect that only he understood.

Ian was put in the heated pool. But as he had never learnt to swim he had no idea of what he should be doing. (Time and again he was helped in his recovery by knowing from his pre-neuropathy experience.) When he tried to stand up in the water he could not see his body and limbs properly. Nor could he feel the bottom. He stubbed his toes on the floor and came out with bleeding splintered toe nails. It was one of the less successful experiments and was not repeated.

The good ideas far outnumbered the bad, however. For a morning he would bend and unbend a paper clip, learning to use his fingers, with his eyes for feedback. He learnt to catch with sandbags, and to build up strength with spring-loaded devices he could pull and push under visual control. He did simple gardening for hours on end.

Yvonne Moir's technique was comparatively simple in approach:

'I would say, "Now we will *stand up*." You have to be positive about what you do, because people, especially the handicapped, rarely think they can get to the next stage. At first with Ian you could see the look of terror on his face when you suggested something new. But as long as you protect the patients, you can carry it through. Sure he often fell, but each time we picked him up.'

They had to, because at least in the beginning he could not have got up by himself. Dozens of times he fell onto the hard wooden floor. He was just picked again. He was often terrified, but he never refused to have a go and used to say to himself: 'To try and fail is understandable, to refuse to try is unforgivable.'

With the illness he had lost not only the ability, but also the desire, to write and draw. At Odstock he began to use a pencil again. Propped up in a chair at a table, he practised and practised. In occupational therapy they helped him with basic writing patterns, using built-up pens and pencils. Their aim was to keep him continually doing the same sort of things with slightly different presentations. Board games like solitaire in scaled-up versions provided a relief from the paper-clip or pen. It didn't really matter what the task was, as long as he kept at it, trying to recover the ability to use hands and fingers.

*

In physiotherapy the emphasis was on building up muscles connected with walking or kneeling, but in occupational therapy the accent was more on skills. Manipulatory movements like writing depend crucially on feedback from the eyes and hands. Ian needed to spend hours evolving alternative techniques of eye-hand co-ordination in order to pick up and manipulate small objects. If he could see no way of performing a task he would think of a way of circumventing it. He couldn't turn over the page of a book. So, as we have seen, he evolved a way of licking his finger and sticking a page to it. That is also how he picked up pieces of the innumerable jigsaw puzzles. His time was spent repeating movement tasks day after day and devising new ways of approaching problems. Once he wrote a letter and licked the stamp to put on the envelope. But then he lost the stamp on his tongue and, not having any feeling in the fingers, couldn't locate it in his mouth. By the time he did scrape it off his tongue it was a useless soggy mess. Ever since he has always licked the envelope and placed the stamp on it.

Interestingly enough, drawing came back before writing. Soon astonishingly controlled drawings began to appear. Someone said that Ian's drawing skills were unaffected by the neuropathy, though it is difficult to imagine and no examples of his pre-illness drawing remain.

He also began to write poetry. But the poems, often composed during long evenings of reflection, tended to express his pessimism about the future. Though the new atmosphere and the enthusiasm of his therapists had had their effect, underneath Ian remained unconvinced of real achievement. He usually destroyed the poems, just as he made his mother destroy all photographs of him in a wheelchair. But one poem remains from this time. What is striking, apart from the fact that it obviously originates in his work experience, is its equation of lack of movement with lack of life. This at a time when he was denied all purposeful movement, though he had normal motor nerves and muscles, because they were deprived of their necessary sensory feedback. We should also realise, however, that Ian tended to write when he felt at his lowest, and the pessimism was not therefore a continuous or even perhaps a dominant mood.

He worked at drawing and writing, but perhaps most of all at standing. Five days a week he would try various things with the help of the therapists, and when they went home he would keep trying back in the hostel. His rate of progress might appear slow, but to the

Living Death

Turned every two hours
Like a joint of meat.
Basted with lotions.
Unmoving like a statue,
Mind filled with emotion.
Limbs dead to the touch,
Movement impossible.
Lying on a bed eyes fixed
On a flaking ceiling.
Wishing those flakes
Would turn to cracks,
And the ceiling fall,to
Take me from this misery.
What use an active brain
Without mobility.

Figure 5. 'In the early days at Odstock one of the doctors asked me to have a go at writing, both as something to do and to give him some feedback on my thoughts and feelings. I was totally frustrated with the typewriter, which seemed to have a mind of its own. After correcting it a few times, I couldn't be bothered to correct the misalignment.'

medical staff it was astonishingly fast given his level of disability. An assessment after six weeks noted:

> Standing 5-10 minutes
> Walking with aid (frame or on parallel bars)
> Can stand on knees and catch balls and hit balls
> Some writing now with a thick pen, now legible

A week later:

> We should try to get him to walk on elbow crutches. This may prove more difficult than he thinks.

After standing at wall-bars, he had progressed to standing without holding on and to taking steps in parallel bars. He often fell, and he had to learn to fall correctly. To fall tensely was to risk greater injury and pain, and once he hurt his back. There was a big difference between balancing when stationary and when moving. In even the smallest movement we make hundreds of unconscious postural adjustments to keep ourselves in the best position. We realise this if we injure a part and try to move without pain. Bell put it thus:

> We may demonstrate upwards of fifty muscles of the arm and hand, all of which must consent to the simplest action; but this gives an imperfect view of the extent of the relation of parts which is necessary to each act of volition. We are most sensible to this combination in the muscles, when inflammation has seized any of the great joints of the body: for even when in bed, every motion of an extremity gives pain, through the necessity of a corresponding movement in the trunk. When we stand, we cannot raise or extend the arm without a new position of the body, and a poising of it, through the action of a hundred muscles.

Ian discovered all this the hard way. If he moved one leg forward but did not move his centre of gravity forward, or counterbalance one movement with another, he would fall.

'If someone said reach for something I knew I couldn't simply do it but had to move an arm and then a leg in the opposite way to compensate.'

He had to concentrate on every part of every movement, with its consequence for balance and for the next movement. Once he had learnt one trick he would pass on to the next, but it must not be assumed that he built up a memory for certain movements. No motor

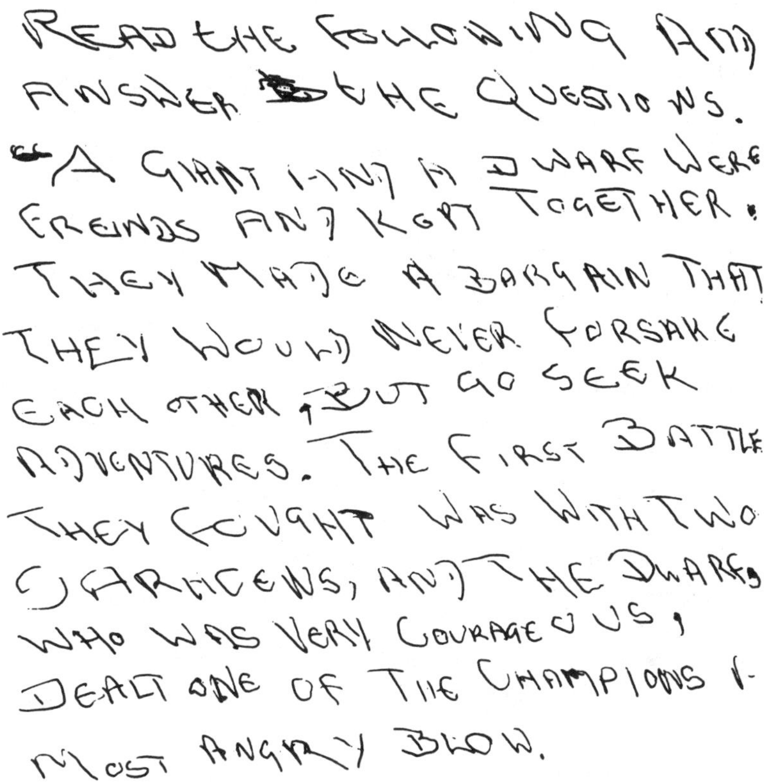

READ THE FOLLOWING AND
ANSWER THE QUESTIONS.
"A GIANT AND A DWARF WERE
FRIENDS AND KEPT TOGETHER.
THEY MADE A BARGAIN THAT
THEY WOULD NEVER FORSAKE
EACH OTHER, BUT GO SEEK
ADVENTURES. THE FIRST BATTLE
THEY FOUGHT WAS WITH TWO
SARACENS, AND THE DWARF,
WHO WAS VERY COURAGEOUS,
DEALT ONE OF THE CHAMPIONS A
MOST ANGRY BLOW.

Figure 6. The earliest example of Ian's handwriting after the neuropathy. Note the letters are written differently at different times (for example the letter A). 'In writing there were not and still are not any suitable movements from the fingers. The pen is gripped tightly between the thumb and the side of the curled up first finger. All movement comes from the wrist.'

act has ever not required conscious awareness. As his repertoire increased, so did the concentration required.

'This need to concentrate was total. I cannot emphasis enough the effort needed to build up in my mind every move and counter move.'

He often fell and often turned over an ankle, partly because his ankles were weak through disuse but partly because there was no feedback. The ankle joint's stability depends to a great extent on feedback from its various ligaments and muscles. Often a ligament is torn and mends but the proprioceptive nerves don't recover completely, and the ankle never fully regains its own stability. For this reason Ted Cantrell suggested a calliper for support, but Ian refused. It would have been a sign of disability, and Ian reasoned as before that once the ankle was artificially braced it would never recover its strength and integrity. By now he was becoming happier to discuss things with his doctors and physiotherapists. Cantrell was wise enough to know that patients should become experts in their own problems, and indeed encouraged it.

The hospital notes show that Ian's attitude had become more positive:

'When I went to Odstock my parents went through a really bad patch and were splitting up. I had no security there. I had no desire to stay in hospital, though I realised the comforts and dangers of institutionalisation. I couldn't go back to being a butcher. So what could I do? But I also began to feel that I was improving. I was becoming more honest with myself and reconciled to my illness. I realised I had to become independent.'

At Christmas he couldn't have entertained the thought of independence, let alone of walking.

As Ted Cantrell had suggested, standing with bars or with help was one thing, but walking without bars would prove far more difficult. At first he graduated to walking behind a frame, or behind a wheelchair with a physiotherapist to help. He had been complaining about the hard wooden floors for months and had got to know nearly every plank face to face. He had been asking to go outside so long that eventually they agreed.

'I remember some time after I'd been at Odstock I went out on to one of the lawns with a physio. I'd moaned about the floors, which were full of splinters. So we walked round and round this lawn, and she said, "You're doing great. I'm just going inside." I'm left holding on to a wheelchair feeling fairly safe but I could only walk round or stand. I was OK standing, but then it began to rain, and I hadn't enough confidence to get up a step and open a door. So I just stayed there getting wetter and wetter until they remembered and came to get me.'

Though by now he was walking behind a wheelchair, all

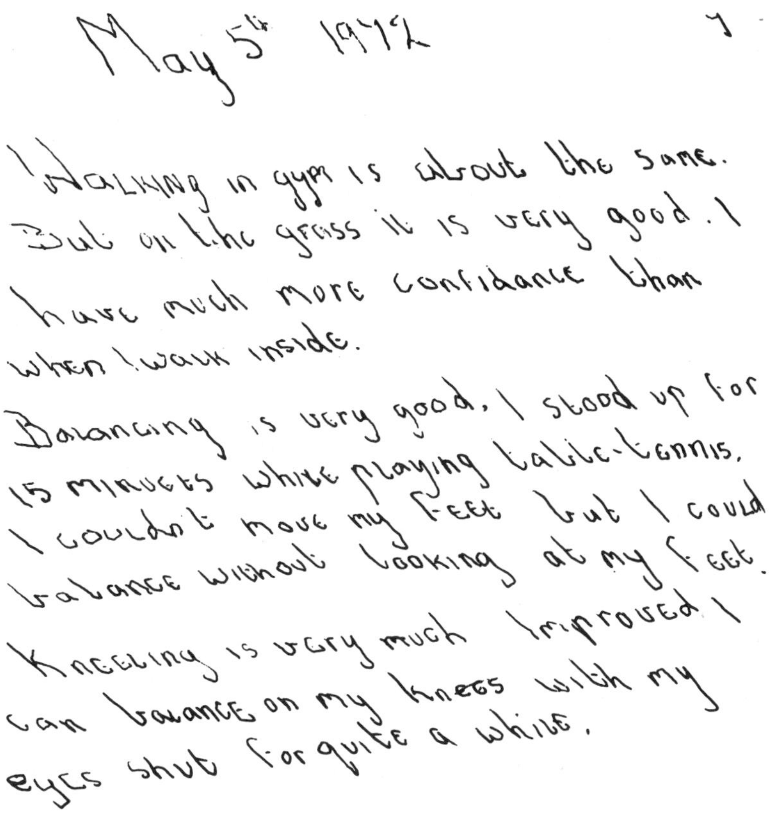

May 5th 1972

Walking in gym is about the same. But on the grass it is very good. I have much more confidance than when I walk inside.

Balancing is very good. I stood up for 15 minutes while playing table-tennis, I couldn't move my feet but I could balance without looking at my feet.

Kneeling is very much improved. I can balance on my knees with my eyes shut for quite a while.

Figure 7. Ian's handwriting two months later. A large improvement, with small letters and much more reproducibility of individual letters.

movements had to be performed under visual control and attended by absolute concentration. Ian's new way of walking couldn't be mistaken for the old. To keep his balance he had to have his feet widely separated on the ground. He could not allow his knees to bend either; otherwise the legs collapsed. In fact his whole body was immensely stiff both in standing and walking, which added to the exhaustion. To avoid dragging his foot on the floor as the leg moved forward he lifted it out by his side high into the air, and without proprioception dropped it hard down in front of him on the heel. It was jerky, tense and slow. He advanced like a wooden puppet activated by a novice, and in a way that's exactly what he was.

The great Russian neuropsychologist A.R. Luria, after Head, often used the term 'kinetic melody',[4] to describe the movements of walking, dancing and running.[5] Music has long been associated with marching and dance. Luria showed how the act of walking or running may be seen as melodic in its smooth and apparently effortless sliding from one phase to the next. This connection between motion and music may be puzzling when applied to normal people, though to see a child running and skipping along, unaware of the world, does suggest music.[6] But the musical analogy begins to seem more substantial when the kinetic melody is destroyed by neurological disease. The hemiplegic gait of a stroke victim, or the slowed, hunched, cramped gait of a Parkinsonian patient, shows how clearly disease can abolish this musical flow of movement. With his loss of muscle tone at rest and his stiff jerky movements when walking, Ian had not only lost his kinetic melody but was also atonal: a twentieth-century man.

*

As he gained confidence, so he began to fit in with the other men in the unit. They worked out a division of labour for the chores, though they soon let Ian know he was not expected to take part. He had tried drying up after meals but kept smashing things. He felt he wasn't pulling his weight, but he had to accept strangers doing things for him.

They had some good laughs as they all struggled to find a place in the world. One patient used to snore loudly. Fortunately he never slept long, but that caused another problem: at night he would keep his light on, to the great annoyance of the others. One night the man in the next bed could stand it no longer and started swearing. The snorer disappeared to the kitchen and everyone went back to sleep. They were woken by a terrible burning smell. In the half-light Ian could see the snorer sitting up under a dimmed light, with smoke trailing up from his shade. He had gone to the kitchen, made a paste from Bisto and smeared it all over his light bulb. Not only did he snore but he apparently had no sense of smell.

One friend, Mark, used to have a girlfriend in Salisbury and go AWOL to spend the night with her. He would come back first thing in the morning on a staff bus so that he could have breakfast back in the ward. To avoid any problems he would put a mop and pillow in his bed for the night in case there was a head count. This worked well until a cleaner arrived early one morning and wanted to know where her mop was. The boys directed her to Mark's bed. She never saw the funny side of finding her mop asleep in a bed.

Larry was a very straight guy with little sense of humour who only had deep and meaningful conversations, a 'brain cell on legs'. 'One day he was in physio on a mat doing press-ups to strengthen his injured arm. He was about half way through when I told him he was wasting his time. "Why?" he asked. "Well," I said, "perhaps you've not realised it yet, Larry, but your girl friend left five minutes ago." He carried on for a couple more press-ups before collapsing. No one had seen him laugh before.'

When Ian had arrived he was suspicious and not a little desperate. The doctors, physios and occupational therapists had given him some hope and allowed him see that improvement was possible. His new-found friends in the ward had given him a society to belong to. Within a few months he was beginning to see that there was, after all, a way he could regain a place in the world. The Odstock therapy was working.

6

Sent to Coventry

Odstock's impact on Ian was powerful. For seven months he had been at home, 'a scrap-heap job', having been told there was little to be done; now he was organised five days a week, nine to five, in all sorts of physical activities, surrounded by enthusiastic workers and fellow inmates. For the first time in his life he was part of a small community. He came on, if not in leaps and bounds, at least with an encouraging steadiness.

Did he appreciate the feeling of recovery, of doing things again for the first time since the illness?

'Yes and no. Naturally I was delighted to see improvements, especially after those bleak months at home feeling so isolated. I got a great deal of satisfaction from developing a new trick and overcoming a problem. However, the more I did the more I wanted to do. I was never satisfied with my achievements. I always expected and demanded more of myself. For me it was never a case of finding a level of activity or mobility at which I would be prepared to remain. I always wanted to know the limits of my ability. Having found them, that was where I was going to stay.'

The routine was different each day, but was organised so that he was busy from nine to five. The physical and mental effort was enormous, and at the end of each day, though he never complained, he was tired out. At weekends he would go home to his mother to rest and sleep. Neither Yvonne Moir nor Kathy Fielding, his occupational therapist, remember Ian saying how tired he was from all the exertion. If they had known they might have eased up a little, but there again it was important to maintain momentum. Seeing improvement was its own motivation, both for Ian and the staff.

After three months he could stand for forty minutes on crutches and walk the length of the parallel bars. One might think it tedious just to stand; but Ian never 'just stood'. All the time he was concentrating, bracing his back, keeping each leg straight, stopping his ankles from turning over. Whether moving or standing, he was concentrating so much that he didn't have time to be bored.[1]

The physios were so pleased with his progress that they thought there must have been some neurological recovery. A visit to Dr Graveson in Neurology Out-patients was arranged.

Ian had waited a long time for this moment: to go back to the man who had said he would never walk again and not be wheeled in but walk. He sat outside in the waiting area, chatting to some of the nurses he had known while he was in the Centre. They were genuinely pleased and enthusiastic about his progress. Ian was so happy to have impressed them. Next, he was thinking, would be Dr Graveson.

'I remember walking into his consulting room on my elbow crutches and standing before his desk thinking, "There you are, you old bugger. What have you got to say now?"

'He just peered over the top of his glasses and offered me a seat. "Hello, Ian. Good to see you." Not a word about "Well done. Bloody great to see you standing", or "I didn't realise you were so tall." Nothing! He went through the usual tests and scribbled his notes. Then with his usual "Fine, see you in six months" I was out in reception. Competent neurologist he may have been, communicator he was not. I quite liked him really, but he was definitely of the old school. It would have taken more than me walking to get him excited.'

On formal neurological examination no recovery had taken place in the nerves, making his improvement all the more astonishing. Ian was improving solely and literally by his own effort. Yet, as far as he can remember, Dr Graveson asked nothing about how he was managing to walk, or what tricks he was using to do all the things Dr Graveson had said he would never do again. It confirmed Ian in his view that his doctors had no understanding of, or real interest in, his condition or its consequences.

'Anyway, I had proved him wrong, and childish though it may have been, it pleased me enormously.'

The motivational power of proving someone wrong shouldn't be underestimated. Ian was fighting for his independence and self-esteem. But we are necessarily social animals, and to some extent we judge ourselves and our performance in relation to others and to the expectations others have of us. To confound a prediction is irrefutable evidence of improvement and worth. Perhaps that is one reason why we are keen to prove others wrong. Such a prediction also gives us something to aim at, and sometimes goals are better provided for us by others than by ourselves. Anyway the motivational power of 'proving the buggers wrong' played a considerable part in Ian's rehabilitation. Time and again he set out to exceed people's expectations and do something they said couldn't be done. This isn't of course to suggest that such a technique should be used intentionally by doctors and physiotherapists, but it would be equally unfair not to mention that Ted Cantrell was well aware of such effects.

*

A nephew, Paul, was born soon after Ian's illness. Ian and his brother laid a bet as to who would walk first, and soon a race was on. Paul walked at about twelve months, and Ian just won. That, however, was not at all to the liking of Ian's niece Natalie. She burst out crying the first time she saw Uncle Ian walk. She had known him over a year, and he had not stood up before. The surprise of seeing him do it unnerved her.

*

In parallel with the physical training, Dr Cantrell was chipping away trying to improve Ian's intellectual aspirations. He realised that Ian would need to support himself and that he could no longer do a manual job. He therefore began to suggest some academic pursuits. Ian readily admits how resistant he was to this and what a hard time he gave Ted Cantrell. At 19 few youths are keen on doctors, especially doctors who keep talking about going back to school, which Ian had loathed. 'It's my body, not my mind,' he would plead. Cantrell remembers it as an uphill struggle: arguing, confronting, provoking and cajoling. He suggested a visit to an educational psychologist for an assessment.

It is not difficult to imagine Ian's reaction, but with reluctance and some bad grace he went. The Director of the Rehabilitation Department, Professor Glanville, wrote a letter of introduction: 'He is going to need advice about alternative employment. I have a feeling that he could be roughly classified as a manual non-intellectual, but I hope I am wrong.'

Ian went in to the meeting still protesting that he wasn't going to do an office job, and this dislike of clerical work appeared in the report. The report continued, however: 'Well above average intelligence for learning new things.' He may have hated school, but not through inability.

Dr Cantrell was encouraged to press ahead with ideas for studying, though his approach was gradual and subtly disguised. He played a waiting game, allowing Ian to explore other ideas, knowing all the while that in the end he would have to accept some sort of office job. Physically-demanding jobs were of course out for him so Cantrell concentrated instead on making him into an intellectual of some sort. Ian, in fact, graduated from prisoner-of-war novels to books on nature and surprised himself by quite enjoying reading and, dare he say it, reading literature.

*

At this time he was still not quite ready for the demands of employment. His recovery had been surprising, but perhaps only Ian knew how difficult it had been and how demanding it was to maintain:

'Ted Cantrell placed a great deal of emphasis on my obtaining work. It was as though a measure of my rehabilitation was in being able to hold down a steady job. I disagreed with him strongly, and we argued the point often. I was still learning to cope with my disability. It was early days, and the concentration required was exhausting. I didn't feel at the time that I could cope with all the mental effort involved in being mobile and in having a job. I was annoyed by the constant pushing in that direction, and I never felt that they accepted my reasons for disagreeing with them. But again I was beaten by the outward signs of my recovery. Again I was convinced that they didn't understand the consequences of my disability. For many disabled people the act of daily living is a job in itself.[2] If they can control their lives that's enough. OK, there are a lot of disabled people who can't manage their own lives, and you must accept that. But many do want to be masters of their destiny, and society should support them. Holding down a job isn't it. Controlling who wipes their behind is.'

Perhaps at times they pushed too hard. With each success more was expected. Often there was an incomplete understanding of how much effort he was putting in and how fragile his recovery was. Once, for instance, he was in the loo and the lights went out. He just sprawled down, completely helpless, and lay there until help arrived.

In many branches of medicine the balance between recovery achieved by the medical staff and recovery achieved by the patient's conscious efforts is tipped in favour of the staff. In pneumonia antibiotics and aids to breathing help the lungs recover even in a patient who cannot help himself. The skilled surgeon does his work when the patient is unconscious. But in rehabilitation there is much more of a balance. The staff work to help the patient recover largely through his own efforts, and the healing process is co-operative. Often it isn't the doctors and paramedical staff who determine the speed of progress but the patient himself. It is the severely brain-damaged patients, who have lost motivation because of their injury, who are difficult or impossible to help because they lack the desire to improve.

Ian sometimes thought that, despite all the wonderful structured help he was given at Odstock, they did not fully appreciate that the improvement was due to him. He may well have been right, especially since the staff had thought at first that his functional recovery was based on a neurological improvement.

*

By September, six months after he had entered Odstock, he was competent at walking with two sticks and could just manage with one. At occupational therapy there were no facilities for meals and the patients had to go across to the canteen two hundred yards away. As soon as he was mobile he insisted on going across on his own, rather than in a wheelchair. His walking was effective but terribly slow. He would set out half an hour before the others, eat and return at the same pace. He was reasonably competent at walking on the flat, but stairs still defeated him. Slopes too were difficult, since he had to lean forward going up and backwards going down. While still learning to keep his body balanced on the flat, he could not learn to lean forward to keep an equilibrium which also depended on forward motion. If he leant to go up a slope and then stopped walking, he would fall forward. It took much thought and experimentation to overcome this problem. Mercifully Odstock's campus was reasonably flat, and the buildings, being huts, had few stairs or ramps.

To be able to walk was, of course, a tremendous boost for his independence and self-esteem. But it had some unforeseen problems. Every advance brought with it an increased risk if anything went wrong. Since he required complete mental concentration, any interruption was disastrous. If he sneezed, he fell over in a heap, and he quickly learnt to sit or lie down until the sneeze had passed. He could not walk and daydream at the same time.

Once, during a weekend break at home, he had tried to show his mother his new ability to walk. He got up from a chair and walked into the middle of the room. Then panic. His limited repertoire only enabled him to stand, sit, or walk a few steps forward. He had not mastered the art of turning to sit in a chair and he needed her help for that. The flat had a hazardous method of electricity supply: by coin-operated meter. When the money ran out, the lights went out. This often happened when Ian was there, and he just fell down where he was. The last time he had just come into the kitchen when Felice was frying up some chips. In falling he narrowly missed the boiling fat pan. After that they changed the meter and paid quarterly.

It was good to have brothers too. One of them soon devised a scheme to keep Ian in his place if he got too cocky. If Ian was standing, he would throw a towel on to his feet and shout, 'Get out of that then!' Unable to see what he was standing on, Ian was helpless and had to tumble over. The brothers may not have had a sound knowledge of the problem, but they soon discovered its effects, and they had a wickedly playful sense of humour.

Once they had him upright, the physiotherapists did not just try to improve his walking, but had him playing table-tennis and, when he sat down, throwing footballs around. As with children, much learning took place in play. The reaching and moving involved taught him consciously to make compensatory postural adaptations. With a similar aim he was made to stand up or kneel, and deliberately bumped into, so he would know how to cope when he left the hospital.

Within a few months of going to Odstock his writing became legible. Though an exacting task, it was less difficult, say, than walking, which involved concentration upon many more sets of muscles acting across many more joints. His writing had changed quite markedly since the illness. The first time he tried to cash a cheque at his bank they refused to accept it, and he had to see the manager to explain, or try to explain, what had happened.

*

One day he was sitting in rehabilitation and glanced up at the wall. There was an unusual picture, apparently in wood, and he asked what it was. It was an example of marquetry: the cutting, inlaying and lacquering of tiny pieces of different sorts of wood to form a design. Whoever explained it to Ian had the temerity to add: 'You can't do it. You'd have all your fingers off.'

It was a foolish thing to say.

'Now I have always liked wood, and the picture I had seen particularly impressed me. I had lots of spare time, and with the added incentive of proving I could do it, I gave it a go. It took ages to cut the pieces required for the picture, but eventually I mastered it. An added bonus was that it was tremendously effective in helping me regain some sort of dexterity. With no feedback through my usual senses I learnt to rely on sight and sound. I learnt the need to plan each stage meticulously. As much as anything it was a great mental exercise.'

The pieces of wood were thin and delicate, and sometimes incredibly small. To cut them, or chisel them, and then stick them down into a pattern was an intricate job requiring great patience. Like the jigsaw puzzles, Ian had chosen almost instinctively to do something, which though it was play, would force him to improve manipulation, the neurological function most dependent on the peripheral proprioceptive function he had lost. Could he have thought of anything more difficult?

'No. At first I used kits, still having to cut and shape the wood, but with a set design to build up. Then I progressed to design my own. It certainly kept my mind occupied – looking at a small piece of wood, working out where to split it without letting it splinter and where it was going to go, both once I had split it and once I had I found it again in the design. Apart from the technicalities of marquetry, I had to work out how I was going to do it, literally – how much pressure I had to put on to a knife to cut a given piece of wood. I learnt by trial and error that, say, wenge is a hard wood and sycamore and chestnut softer. You find out by seeing and hearing. You get a feel for it – well, if not a feel, at least an understanding. I broke many many pieces of wood reaching that stage.'

In fact, while at Odstock, and when he was at his mother's at weekends and during occasional holidays, he would sit for hours in a chair propped up doing marquetry. By this time Felice had gone back to work. She remembers leaving him at the table in the morning and he would still be there in the evening when she came back. The floor would be covered in small chippings and discarded shards of wood, and on the table would be the few, often very few, pieces considered good enough to take their place in the design.

What he produced wasn't just examples of marquetry such as a child might bring home from school, but beautifully finished pieces of elaborate design. As in other things, his motive was to be compared with able-bodied people. He even sold a couple of pictures, and thought of trying to make them for a living. Mercifully he decided he could not produce the work quickly enough for that. In any case, as he says, there was no real point carrying on with it since he had proved to himself, and others, that he could do it. The precious time and mental energy could be put to better use.

*

Ted Cantrell continued to drop his small depth-charges in Ian's mind about the need to think about employment. It was difficult. Ian had done so much just to become physically independent. To have to consider a job as well, and with it the loss of his place in the hostel, was too much as yet. This and the probability of living alone in a bedsit was hard to contemplate. It was made even harder because he had lost the ability to do the only thing that had really engaged him, butchering.

He entertained various ideas, only to drop them. For example, he thought of working with animals or with handicapped children. Dr Cantrell realised the impracticality of many of these ideas but bided his time until Ian came to the same conclusion. Ian suggested becoming an architectural draughtsman – an astonishingly bold idea given the nature of his handicap. It was arranged that he should see round an architect's studio and talk to a draughtsman. Fortunately nothing came of it. Probably his complete lack of qualifications led him to discount it. Despite Ian's oft-stated hatred of offices, Cantrell could see that that was where he was inevitably headed. Since he would eventually have to accept it, Ted just let him exhaust the other possibilities.

Whatever career was finally chosen, qualifications were a necessary start. Studying would also provide a new challenge, and Ian was ready for that. An attempt was made to enrol him at the local college to take three 'O' levels. But it was difficult to get in. It wasn't that the academic requirements were too high, but that the main entrance to the college was at the top of a flight of steps through a set of heavy glass doors. To add to the problem, building work was being carried out at the front entrance which was a maze of scaffolding and debris. As he could not enter the building by the main entrance he had to resume his education literally by the back door.

It was Ian's first real sortie into the outside world. He had to plan his moves between lectures even more carefully than usual to avoid crowds. His writing was legible but extremely slow. He had learnt to write by holding the pen between his thumb and index finger in a pincer grip. He found it easier to form the letters by moving his elbow and wrist. He could not both attend to lectures and write, so he just listened and made a few notes later when he was back in the hostel.

Though he was pleased to be with the other students he never felt one of them and wasn't completely accepted. One day, towards the end of the course, he overheard one of the students inviting people to a party at her house. He mulled over a good reason for not going but needn't have bothered. He was the only person not asked.

At first he was to take English, History and Sociology, but he soon dropped the last two. He enrolled in the autumn and took the examinations in the summer. Many students seem to regard the writing of exam papers as a speed-writing course, covering as many sheets as possible in the hope that more equals better. For Ian, who had to consider the making of each word (and each letter) consciously, the process was very slow. But despite his evident handicap he refused special allowances, taking his exams in longhand with no extra time: 'No one's going to give me special treatment in the outside world, so I don't want it now.'

The exams were in a gym with the usual canvas sheeting laid to protect the floor, rendering it uncertain and slippery. To find his desk Ian had to wander up and down the rows, and eventually he asked someone to find it for him. The exam went reasonably well, but on his way out he fell. The invigilator came running up to make sure he was all right. Ian just asked if he could have extra marks for sympathy. He passed.

*

Though he was able to walk, it was a slow and ungainly process and involved great effort and risk. For longer distances he had to rely on hospital transport. Public transport presented problems with jerky rides and sudden braking. The drivers couldn't always be relied on to be aware of the special needs of the handicapped. Once, a friend of Ian's with cerebral palsy, who was just able to walk but used his wheelchair for longer distances, was waiting by a bus stop and when the bus came got out of the chair to enter. The driver took the fare and drove off, leaving the wheelchair waiting at the bus stop!

The obvious solution was for Ian to drive himself. Most important, he had learnt to drive before his illness and already had a provisional licence. A letter of application for a hand-controlled invalid carriage was sent to the appropriate Board of Assessment: 'With his eyes closed,' said the report, 'he has little idea of where his limbs are in space...but we do not necessarily want to deny him the opportunity to drive.' In fact Ian had been driving a machine surreptitiously round the hospital without much problem. A further letter was sent a few weeks later, before he was assessed. Someone had realised that at night Ian might not be able to see his hands. In practice, however, this wasn't a problem and Ian passed the audition. He had a single stick control, like a tiller, for steering, accelerating and braking. It was relatively easy to retain the stick in his field of vision while keeping an eye on the road. He did not really need to look at the controls, because to some extent he could use feedback from the scene outside. This is more or less the way able-bodied people drive. They don't think, 'I'll press my foot down so much to increase speed', but judge how fast the car is going by the passage of scenery.

Even if the machine was, in his words, 'a battery-driven biscuit tin', to be independently mobile was important for Ian, as it is for many disabled people. Life in the fast lane wasn't without its troubles, however. In traffic jams and slow-moving traffic, judging his movement from the motion of things around him, he often had difficulty knowing whether it was he who was moving or the next line of cars. This double-take happens to us all at times, but it was compounded for Ian because he had no information about posture and locomotion from the sensitive receptors of joint angles and skin pressure. That he had this difficulty despite a normal inner-ear apparatus for balance suggests that perception of movement and orientation depends not only on vision and the inner ear but also on proprioceptive clues from our joints and ligaments.[3] In aircraft, when the visual clues are removed, we depend not only on the ear to tell us of motion and uprightness but also on the subtle information coming from receptors in our skin and joints. In a plane Ian is badly disoriented.

Sitting in the 'biscuit-tin' was better than dependence on others, but if anything went wrong Ian was helpless. If he had a flat tyre or a mechanical failure, he had to get out and stand by the roadside waving for help. Sometimes passing motorists would smile and wave back, saying to themselves, as Ian put it, 'Look, dear. There's a cripple waving. Wave back!'

The battery-driven carriage only had a range of 20-40 miles and so was not very practical for the countryside where distances are greater. Nor was it very fast. One day Ian was going up the steep hill from Odstock to the downs. He swears he was overtaken by a woman on foot pushing a pram. After that he asked for a petrol-engined model, which some time later they gave him.

*

Now that he was walking, dressing and feeding himself and was mobile, Ian had less need to stay in the hostel and the Rehabilitation

Centre. He had been at Odstock nearly a year, and Ted Cantrell suggested he should live out. But where? Freed from the need to look after him, his mother and father were still together, but everyone encouraged him to find digs for himself in case they split up. Felice planned to live in Jersey, where the facilities for the disabled were less adequate, and he could not live with his father. The only alternative was lodgings. But nothing available seemed quite right.

The doctors and staff grew worried that Ian might become institutionalised and too dependent on the hostel. Ian understood but was in no great hurry to live alone. Once more he had become a victim of his own achievements. The hospital staff, he thought, didn't fully understand the continual effort and vigilance he had to put in. He knew. He knew how hard it was to dress himself and so on, and to study. He could not imagine doing all this *and* the shopping and household chores. He used delaying tactics. But a definite end to his stay in Odstock was in sight.

Hereward College, Coventry, was at that time a fairly new technical college, designed specifically for the disabled. Ted Cantrell and Yvonne Moir had not sent anyone to it before. Ian seemed the ideal guinea-pig. He was willing to try, since he would be able to take his City and Guilds exams and prepare for a clerical job, something he was now resigned to. Besides, he was also keen to have another year shielded from work.

*

So at the end of July 1973 he left Odstock for a brief stay with his family. They even managed a short holiday in Jersey. He had been in the hospital seventeen months, an almost unprecedented period. Yvonne Moir remembers only one other patient who had been there as long. She was a young woman who had suffered a head injury and was quite severely brain damaged. She improved quite markedly once they realised that a large part of her problem was that she had become deaf and taught her to sign.

Ian had arrived 'a scrap-heap job', bitter and not a little angry. When he left, another formal neurological examination showed that there had been no improvement in his neuropathy, but he was able to walk (after a fashion), fend for himself and drive. With Dr Cantrell and the others he had forged a partnership for his rehabilitation. They had given him the correct milieu and support for a new approach to daily living. He had been literally 'put back on his own two feet'. The staff had been able help him develop 'tricks'[4] to circumvent his disability. This had given him a constructive pride in himself. He became more optimistic, and could attempt new movement techniques of his own. As he became more confident he would initiate various physiotherapeutic procedures himself. This of course was good, because only he had a proper knowledge of his unique problem.

Much of his improvement came in the first half of his stay in Odstock. But both Yvonne Moir and Ted Cantrell are quick to point out that it would have been wrong to discharge him as soon as he could feed himself, dress and walk. At that stage he would not have had sufficient confidence or ability to do a job. Their aim was to equip their patients for employment, since that gave them independence and self-esteem. To have taken Ian only half way to that point would have been much less worthwhile. Yvonne Moir concedes that he was there a long time, but she was not surprised: 'At that time we were able to respond to the need. We were particularly keen to get people placed in work if at all possible, rather than just to reach a plateau in either physiotherapeutic or OT terms. Placing them in work gives them a station in life independent of their disability. It's a whole-person thing, rather than just trying to chart their physical progress.'

Ted Cantrell agrees: 'The length of time people were taken was determined by themselves and by their progress. We tended to take people until they stopped improving. Ian continued to improve. He had failed at school and came from a failed family, though he had a splendid mother. We had to try to help him not only to recover physically but to gain enough resilience and self-respect to be independent. I'm still not quite sure how he managed to stay so long, but it all takes time. Most patients seem to run into a brick wall. I've often seen patients with strokes, for example, recover so much and then say, unconsciously, "That's enough." They may have done more at one time than they settle for at the end.'

It is as though having explored the full extent of their recovery, people prefer to live within their limitations, even if it means retreating slightly into their physical disability. This of course is not unique to the disabled; few able-bodied people like to have to do their best every day. When the disabled reach this plateau, beneath the summit, everyone knows, from patient to physiotherapist to doctor. The end point has been reached. With Ian that didn't happen because he kept improving and wanting to do more. He was prepared both to explore the limits of his disability and to continue to live at these limits.

On his arrival the team had concluded that he would probably improve his movement skills so as to regain some independence and take a job in, say, an office suitable for a young man in a wheelchair. Yvonne Moir soon changed her mind. She began to think he would walk and live independently. So why didn't the doctors think so too? Why were they so gloomy? 'They may well have been more knowledgeable and realistic than me,' she said. ' I could have been wrong. But I still hold to my theory that if patients have a good brain they can overcome physical disability. Intellectually, Stanley Graveson couldn't see that someone with Ian's disability could walk. I couldn't see how grave his disability was, but I couldn't conceive that with his mind he wouldn't recover. If you haven't been through an experience before, you have no idea where to go. Though we hadn't seen it before either, we just got on with it.'

It would take a brave man, doctor or patient, to disagree. Her encouragement and enthusiasm tended to make her predictions self-fulfilling.

Refusing to accept Ian's plea that it was his body not his mind, Ted Cantrell and the physios set about retraining body and mind together so that he could stand up in, and to, the world. Ian took some persuading, but they got there in the end. His gratitude is complete.

7

Skinning a Cat

Ian was driven up to Coventry by a Social Services driver. His electric tricycle obviously did not have sufficient range for the journey. Hereward College was purpose-built for the disabled and seemed ideal. The accommodation block and lecture rooms were all on one site, so travelling around was no problem. Ian settled into his shared room. Everything was custom-built, and for most of the inmates it was a marvellous place. But Ian soon found it soulless. Perhaps, after nearly two years in a hut with his mates, anywhere would seem have seemed so, but he did not feel at ease.

He was disappointed to discover that many of the lecturers were not very approachable. Having come from a place where communication and team spirit were key factors, he found the environment too rigid. Ted Cantrell and Yvonne Moir had been open-minded and had encouraged patient participation in decision-making, to develop independence. At Hereward the attitude was the opposite. The administration tried to run the site on strict lines, and Ian began to wonder whether he had made the right decision going there. To be cautious, he changed his course from 'O' level to office studies. This gave him the option of a two-year business course or, after his first year, of ending with a piece of paper which would give him a foot in the door of an office. Lectures were compulsory. If you did not attend you were asked why, and you had to produce a good reason. Many of the people there had been disabled from birth and were completely institutionalised. That may have been why the staff shepherded them so much. But Ian could not help thinking that they might have relaxed things here, of all places, and allowed some liberty. For instance, one day there were arguments and threats by the staff when a student was told not to wear a hat in the canteen at mealtimes:

'I couldn't believe it. They hounded this chap for ages trying to get him to take his woollen hat off at mealtimes. They said it was unhygienic, anti-social and disrespectful. Can you see this type of administration surviving in an ordinary college for the same age-group? I'm sure I couldn't. You see, the administration and some of the lecturers came from schools which dealt with disabled infants and they tried to run Hereward on the same lines. The students who had been in institutions for years didn't seem to mind, but those who had been used to a bit of freedom and self-expression, and those who had been to ordinary colleges, found it all too much. To my mind it didn't attempt to fulfil the important role of colleges of preparing people for the outside world. In that respect Hereward failed abysmally.'

The petty rules were operated even outside lectures. For instance, showers were not allowed after 10.30. One night there was a fire drill at 11. One fellow came out clad in a towel and dripping wet. The supervisor asked if he had been having a shower, 'Oh no, I just sweat a lot in bed.'

There was a canteen so that they did not have to prepare their own meals. It was a pity the food was so awful. Once Ian had a beefburger served up with its wrapper still on; cucumbers covered in mould were not uncommon. Another disadvantage for Ian was that he couldn't carry his tray from the hatch to the tables and had to get someone else to do it. He still hated having his disability paraded in public.

The office studies course included machine accounting, business accounting and typewriting. None of these subjects enthralled him, but he was a reliable student. He still hated academic study, but the deal was clear. If he could get through the course he would be able to find a job in the real world in a year or two. Even he could master that equation.

*

He got on fine with most of his fellow students. But he found that some of them had the wrong attitude. When they discussed their plans for the future, it became obvious that many were professional students who regarded study in Coventry as an end in itself. They didn't expect to find a job when their time at Hereward was over, but rather to go on leading the same lives as before. For Ian this was heresy. For him the purpose of study was to gain qualifications to allow him, if not to escape from the disabled world, at least to be better equipped to compete outside. Many of the others seemed to have accepted that world and to be using Hereward as a two-year intellectual holiday-camp. They were happy with the restrictive rules, since the staff were only trying to make life easier for the students. He began lose sympathy with many of the staff and some of the students. He felt like McMurphy in *One Flew Over the Cuckoo's Nest*.

Ian was different from most of the others. His disability was comparatively recent and he wanted to return to the real world as soon as possible, a journey not possible for many of his fellows. Yet he was liked by the others. He was always keen to help and was ready with a smile and a joke when any one was feeling low. He soon gained their respect and was the natural man to be made social committee chairman. He was put in charge of the students' bar on the rare occasions it was allowed to be open. He was ideal for this because he could not drink much, since if he did he became too unsteady to function.

Some of the students would go out in the evenings, and at weekends they explored hostelries in the countryside. Long Indian files of disabled trikes were assembled to crawl along country lanes in search of pubs with good beer and no steep steps. Ian would ride at the back as shot-gun, ready to attend to stragglers or breakdowns.

He soon learnt to manipulate his position as social committee chairman and, when organising outings frequently arranged them at a time when the college driver was booked for an official trip: that is, when the bus was being used by the staff. Then, as the administration had specified in their prospectus that 'adapted transport would be available for social outings', the staff would have to provide theirs at their own expense. Sometimes he was hauled up before the Principal to discuss these double bookings. But there was nothing they could do. For his part he enjoyed kicking against the establishment. He had tried at Odstock – but, damn it, Ted Cantrell had been too nice to upset for long.

It was not only lectures that were compulsory: everyone had to do art. One man with severe cerebral palsy refused, saying he wanted qualifications not drawings. Ian could see his point. So many disabled people had such difficulty with any kind of movement that concentration on tasks they considered irrelevant was a shameful waste of mental energy. They hounded this poor fellow until he gave in. Like Ian he had been interested in wood, and he asked to do wood-turning. They refused on grounds of safety. So in the end he did not do art and nobody won. Ian disliked the way they hounded the man with their rules. Worse, they had shown their lack of true understanding of what it was like to be disabled.

The courses were primarily academic but included some tests on motor skills. In one of these a perfect circle had to be cut from a piece of paper with scissors. Ian used a trick, of course. He folded the paper over into four and cut round one quarter. Then he unfolded it to show a near perfect circle. The teacher gave him full marks. Ian protested that he had cheated, but the teacher would have none of it. The test was the test; nowhere in his instructions was there a clause disqualifying anyone for doing what Ian had done. Ian was furious that he could pass in this way and argued, but it did no good. While others with more dexterity than Ian failed, he passed by trickery.

*

As well as shared rooms, there were also communal kitchens and sitting-out areas. One night they had organised a party, and by the end of it one man who was drunk was sick all over the kitchen. Ian was helping to clear up. It all had to be ship-shape by morning since, if the day-staff had to clear up after parties, the administration would have used such a pretext to ban parties altogether. One of the night-time care assistants, a woman called Lizzie, was helping to clear up. He had seen her before but had never spoken to her, though he wanted to. She was in her early forties, slim and blonde – an older woman many young men would have dreamt of, especially if they had been starved of female company. As they cleared up the mess they got to chatting, and afterwards over a cup of coffee they found, to Ian's surprise, that they had much in common. Not only that. He realised that the attraction was mutual. It was difficult to believe that a beautiful woman like that should find him a turn-on, but it became increasingly clear that she did. It was more than two years since he had touched a woman, and here was a Mrs Robinson figure. He did not need to think about it. He asked her out to the theatre. Soon she invited him round to her house for a meal with her husband and family. Ian was not exactly sure what sort of relationship Lizzie still had with her husband and was reluctant to go at first. But the college food was so awful that the promise of a home-cooked meal was too good to pass up. They soon started an affair.

They would meet late at night in the residence. Since he shared a room they had to go to an empty kitchen or a room not in use. It was handy that she had all the pass keys for the residence and a list of who was away at what time. At first it was all action, and things got very steamy. Though he found that his disability caused some performance problems, that did not seem to matter. There was more than one way to skin a cat, and he delighted in the relationship.[1]

Rumours began to fly. Lizzie went for a weekend break with some of the students and sent Ian a postcard. After that everyone put two and two together. The Principal heard. Though it was not clear what rule they were breaking he tried hard to catch them misbehaving. He even took to prowling round the residence late at night. But they were much too canny and kept one step ahead. Outwitting him added to the excitement and eventually he gave up. Once Ian fell asleep during a lecture. The teacher made some comment about too many late nights with care attendants.

He didn't mind. After so long it was good to have a relationship with any woman, let alone a stunning woman like Lizzie. It did his confidence a power a good. It also enhanced his credibility with the other students. What he never understood was what went on between Lizzie and her husband, especially when the husband started turning up to help him run the bar.

*

At the end of his first year there were exams. Ian was asked if he would like extra time but again refused. He managed to pass without difficulty, gaining credits in all but two subjects. Then he had to decide whether to carry on with the next year or quit after one year with the minimal qualifications for an office job. The work was going well and, what with Lizzie and his other social activities, he had certainly spread his wings. But he was still unhappy as a student and wanted to try the world outside. At the end of the summer term they all said their goodbyes and looked forward to seeing him in the autumn term. He said nothing, but he was not convinced he would return.

He spent that summer at home with his family and took a short break with his aunt and uncle in Jersey. Slowly he reached the decision not to go back to Coventry. He would try his luck in a job instead. Lizzie wrote to him once or twice, but there was no future in their relationship, as they both realised.

In the year at Hereward his confidence had increased. But for the most part he had been segregated with other disabled people and so had been perceived as disabled himself. After being among able-bodied students in Salisbury, he was unhappy at being separated from them. It was that particularly he wanted to leave behind. This McMurphy left Hereward intact and with a few memories of the battles he had won against the Miss Ratchets.

But Coventry's approach had merit. At that time Ian had a struggle just to move around in any society. Given that, it is doubtful whether he could have managed to be in a conventional college and been able to enjoy all the educational benefits and opportunities. Yvonne Moir points to another example:

'In Salisbury there is still a grammar school, and it is very good. One disabled boy was considered "too bright" to go away to a school for the disabled, and so for his intellectual advancement he was sent to the grammar. It was a disaster. As the only disabled boy, the other boys, even the schoolmaster, were beastly to him. Eventually he went away to a special school. It made all the difference to his confidence and self-esteem as well as to his academic work. It wasn't that he couldn't cope with the grammar school, it was that school society couldn't cope with him.'

How different from the marvellous story of Joseph in Christopher Nolan's *Under the Eye of the Clock*.

'Ian may be right,' said Yvonne. 'People should be allowed choices. But that choice may allow "normal" people to be nasty to the disabled. In handicapped schools, handicapped children are very good and kind to each other. Put them in a normal school and their attitude is not the same.'

Disabled people are individuals like anyone else, and their needs vary.[2] In an ideal world schools should be flexible enough to take that into account. But in the world as it is, Hereward did its best for its students and, when all was said and done, did pretty well for Ian.

*

Ian spent the year in Coventry trying to escape from his ghetto of disability. By the end of his time there he had passed the examinations and was ready to rejoin the human race and the rat race. Yet despite his efforts to relearn movements his repertoire and daily routines remained very different from other people's. All movements still had to be under conscious control and continuous visual inspection. Without thought there was no movement. His actions for the day, for any day, reflected his thoughts for the day. These thoughts were the result of nearly three years' experimentation: three years of thinking all day, every day – thinking how to get by while still having some mental energy available to do more than just get by, for he wanted not just to function but to live.

For instance, Ian slept on his back, or slightly to one side. To lie on his front was difficult, because he could not see his body, and if he could not see it he could not move it. If he lay on his side he ran the risk of lying on an arm and not feeling it at first and then not being able to move it. He always slept with a light on. (I once asked him if he had a torch by the bedside. A stupid question, since he would not be able to see to move in order to find it.)

Most of us, especially in our younger and more exuberant days, have known what it is to wake not knowing where we are. When Ian woke up, his body hidden by bedclothes, he had no idea at first where in the bed he was. Bell had used the knowledge of position in bed for his argument for the 'muscular sense':

> We awake with a knowledge of the position of our limbs: This cannot be from a recollection of the action which placed them where they are; it must therefore, be a consciousness of their present condition. When a person in these circumstances moves, he has a determined effort; and he must be conscious of a previous condition before he can desire a change or direct a movement.[3]

Ian relocated himself in bed in the morning by, say, pushing out a leg. If it became colder, or he felt or heard it bump something, he knew it had moved. If there was no new sensation, it might have become stuck under the other leg. He used clues from the remaining sensations of deep touch and temperature for partial compensation. Often he fell out of bed. As he dropped off to sleep he would have the involuntary jerks we all have. During sleep he would occasionally move quite sharply and might well kick his companion. A further problem, and one which prevented him from sleeping through, was that to turn over he had to wake up. Each time he had to calculate exactly where he was and to do that he had to wake up so much that settling down to sleep again was that much more difficult.

Ian has described how he would sometimes wake to feel a hand on his face and not know to whom it belonged. Until he realised it was his own, the experience was momentarily terrifying. Since he has normal perception of warmth and touch in the face, but only of warmth in the hand, it is interesting that he cannot, or does not, use warmth of the hand alone to identify self from non-self.

He rarely took baths, partly because the bath was slippery and partly because once he was in the water his visual sense of his body was distorted. Manoeuvring in and out presented problems, and sitting down with his legs in front was not a favoured posture. In fact, as many old people find, taking a bath required a fair amount of gymnastic skill. If he had slipped while in the bath, he would have had trouble recovering. He showered instead and bathed only if a shower wasn't available. Baths were mentally demanding. Showers of course were slippery, but less slippery than baths, and he could wedge himself up against a corner. He could never manage with both eyes shut at once, so he had to wash his face carefully one side at a time, as in the Camay adverts of the Fifties and Sixties. Hairwashing remained tricky and laborious.

He was able to see to do up buttons on a shirt, and learnt a trick to do up cuff buttons. But he was never able to do up the collar button of a shirt, because he could not see it except in a mirror. Similarly he could knot a tie, but not if he used a mirror. He learnt these fiddly dressing movements, but could not use mirror-reversed visual feedback to guide his fingers. He could use a mirror to comb his hair, but then he has normal touch sensation over the scalp.

He held cups and mugs by their body, not by their handle. He learnt to wait until a hot drink had cooled before taking it, partly in case it was too hot to grasp and partly for fear of spilling it on himself. He worked out never to take a cup from anyone but to ask for it to be put on a flat surface. Then he could check that there was nothing behind it before grasping it. If there was something behind it he had not seen he would be likely to pick it up or knock it over without realising. A full cup, like a clear soup, required far more concentration than a half-full one if it wasn't to be spilt. Plastic or polystyrene cups weren't easy to drink from because of their lack of rigidity. It was difficult to judge how to put enough force into a grasp to hold an object without crushing it.

The list of changed movements was endless: a list that only Ian was aware of. Each activity of daily living posed a different problem to circumvent and overcome. Still, after three years he was ready to take a job and rejoin society. At Odstock he had learnt a sufficient repertoire of movements, and in Coventry he had gained the qualifications. It was like leaving school for a second time – with all the elation, but with the misgivings too. He may have rebelled against Hereward College, but it allowed him a further year to prepare himself. And he could hardly complain about the lack of extra-curricular activities.

8

Coming Alive Again

When he came down from Hereward College Ian went back to live with his family. His mother had decided not to leave. After a few weeks' rest he found a job as a clerical worker in the Civil Service.

Before his formal interview he was required to have a medical, and the doctor chosen for this happened to be Dr Graveson. Ian sat nervously outside his office waiting to go in. The doctor knew his condition as well as anybody and Ian was worried he wouldn't give him the go ahead.

He was led into the office and, as usual, was confronted with the top of Dr Graveson's head, which was kept lowered throughout the interview. Did he think he could cope? What if he was given a task he couldn't manage? What did he think of the hours? Dr Graveson asked the questions and Ian replied to the top of his head.

After a pause Dr Graveson looked up and said: 'Do you really want this job?'

'Yes.'

He stood up, shook Ian by the hand and wished him well.

At the job interview, before a panel of three, he was asked what had happened to him and if he thought he could cope in a big office? Would he need any extra help? Ian answered without too much difficulty. After all, he had been waiting for this interview for several years and wasn't going to allow them to turn him down at this stage. He was taken on, on six months' probation.

Once at work Ian was not so naive as not to expect that some allowances would be made at first for his disability. He immediately ran into problems explaining what was wrong to his colleagues:

'The messages from my hands and feet aren't normal. I can't feel my skin and body properly.'

'But what's that go to do with movement?'

He would explain as best he could, often by analogies: 'You try doing up a shoe-lace with woollen gloves on.' Or, 'It's a bit like when you've been to the dentist. Afterwards you can't feel your lips and so can't drink properly. I'm like that all over my body.' Here the analogy included a physiological event – a nerve blocked by local anaesthetic – so it came a little closer to the truth. It isn't completely accurate, however, since the purpose of a local anaesthetic is to prevent pain, the sensation of which was fortunately preserved in Ian.

The best course, he found, was to get people to ignore the problem while making minor allowances, like not expecting him to carry trays of tea. If someone new appeared he would often say it was his back (with a history of back problems this was a half-lie at worst) and make light of it. Only occasionally did he have to bring people's attention to his problem. For instance, he had to ask, 'Please don't bump into me, because my balance isn't very good.'

He found the office very difficult at first. All the new tricks he had to explore just to do the work physically were quite tiring. Then there was the fact that for eight hours at a time he was in the company of comparative strangers who had little understanding of his condition, and he had to work hard at appearing fairly normal to avoid being stared at. On top of this was the work itself, which required a great deal of care and concentration. It is not surprising that he had little time for anything other than work.

Eventually, though, everything seemed to be settling down and became a little easier. He was earning a living like everyone else. He may have been doing a job that didn't really interest him, but in that he was not alone. His sense of humour played an important part in helping him to overcome these problems and make friends with his colleagues. It was satisfying to reach the stage where he could hold down a job on the same terms as anyone else.

Though his colleagues became friends he didn't see much of them outside work. He soon developed his own hobbies. He bought a proper four-wheeled car. Driving he found both relaxing and enjoyable, for in a car he was as others were and no longer disabled. He did have an orange disabled badge, however, which he usually kept in the boot, along with a set of antlers he had found in the forest. The car had an automatic gearbox and two simple hand controls, one for acceleration and one for braking. They were within his field of vision like the steering wheel, so he did not have to keep looking at them. He rarely used the speedometer, partly because, as we have seen, he judged speed by the visual feedback of the rate at which the surroundings move in relation to the car, and partly because he preferred to ignore it. Driving required far less concentration than walking and was his favourite relaxation.

The opportunity for physical release from the tensions we all feel ('A turn or two I'll walk, to still my beating mind', as Prospero said in *The Tempest*) continued to be denied him. He would often go for a drive to calm himself. The car gave him independence, but it was also a potent symbol of normality when compared with the disabled tricycle. Not just for him either. 'When he was in a three-wheeler,' his brother noted, 'people used to say, "How's your brother?" Now with a car no one asks any more.'

*

In the three years since his illness he had had to be concerned almost exclusively with himself. To return to life, to stand on his own feet had been challenge enough. His motivation had been personal, but he had also delighted in being able to prove all the well-meaning experts, friends and relatives wrong. Such goals lose their power once achieved, yet he had to continue his life.[1] He had striven for three years to reach this stage, without giving much thought to what would happen next.

There's more to life than work, though. The illness had taken him away from his new friends in Jersey and had also taken from him three years. In spite of all his efforts to return to a normal life, he had only returned to the state he had reached on leaving school. He was in a new job. Inevitably he was self-conscious and a little cut off from the others by his condition. What he needed was some simple playful fun. At 22 he wanted a bit more than life at home with the family.

He had been at work for almost nine months and though it wasn't difficult to make friends there he did not see these people out of hours. About this time a letter arrived from a social worker called Jenny, who, together with Pam, a girl he had known in college, was thinking of starting up a group for disabled people in his age group.

His initial reaction was, 'You must be bloody joking.' He had spent years getting away from all that and here was an invitation to become involved in yet another group. But thinking it through and talking to a colleague at work he decided to go to the first meeting.

They met in the flat of a young disabled woman whom Jenny was also attending. Ian had arrived early, and while waiting for the others, they chatted about disabled clubs and their experiences of them. The young woman wasn't particularly keen on the segregated groups either but had gone along with it as a favour to Pam. Eventually Jenny and Pam arrived, followed shortly by Paul, a young man in a wheelchair. Everyone chatted away about whether there was a need for another group. Finally they agreed that there might be a place for one for newly disabled people, where they could meet others with similar problems.

*

At the next meeting Jenny sat next to Ian and a friend of Pam's. Her name was Mavis and she had heard about the meeting from the hospital social worker where she worked. As she had some spare time on her hands she had come along, primarily to offer her services as a secretary.

At eighteen months Mavis had contracted polio. Her elder brother Jim, who was four at the time, remembers little about it, except that their mother screamed with despair. Mavis was taken to the local hospital and then to Lord Mayor Treloar's at Alton, a Regional Centre thirty miles away. As she was paralysed from the neck down her breathing was assisted by a machine, one of the dreaded 'iron lungs.' She was in this for months before the acute effects of the virus receded and she could breathe for herself.

Polio is not a transient disease, and it refused to let her go. The virus eventually passed on, but it left her with a permanent legacy: severe damage to the motor nerves where they begin their path to the muscles in the spinal cord. Her body was left wasted and deformed. She had a weakened and withered right arm and leg, and a severe curvature of the spine. As a child she slowly learnt to use her arms and legs again, though all movement was weak. Being so young, she had hardly begun to perform many of the movements she now had to learn with weakened muscles. She underwent twenty operations to correct the weaknesses. Each one was terrifying. But the damage to the motor nerves of the spinal cord was permanent. Not even the best orthopaedic surgeons, as they changed the alignment of bones and moved tendons, could give her back her muscular strength.

Mavis was in Alton for several years. Her parents had no car and were only able to visit her once a week. In the early 1950s a journey of thirty miles was quite an undertaking especially by public transport. It was also expensive, and the family were not well off. Often, to reduce the cost, they took it in turns to visit. It was only later when her grandfather bought a car which her father was able to borrow that visits became easier.

The hospital authorities didn't allow Jim to visit his little sister and he hardly saw her. Her father would come, kiss her on the cheek and sit at the end of the bed reading the paper, while her mother would be talking about this and that and the other children. They would leave sweets, which were confiscated by the ward nurses and later handed back in rations. Her grandparents lived closer and had more time, so they visited as much they could. But the virus had deprived Mavis of her loving family as surely as it had destroyed her movement.

Despite all this some of her happiness and spirit remained. She would often sing from her hospital bed: at one stage she was given a side ward to herself because she was disturbing the rest of the children. She used to pretend to be asleep when the teachers came round, to avoid the more boring lessons.

Jim remembers his sister returning to the family permanently when he was 10 and she 7. She had a leg calliper and a special corset. She was able to attend a mainstream school but couldn't move about very much. Jim used to carry her round on his back, as did some of her friends. She got on reasonably well, though she had missed so much time that there was no way she could ever catch up.

Her parents found it difficult to cope at times, and for her part Mavis often couldn't understand their concerns. She remembers doing her exercises on a coconut mat each day – Jim would do them too, making it a game. But she always did them in the kitchen rather than in the living room, which was kept for best, and she thought this a snub. In fact they lived without central heating and hot water. Her mother chose the kitchen because it was the warmest room. When they lit a fire in the living room Mavis would exercise in there.

Other memories of her homecoming were happier. Her dad was good at Dad-type things. She loved to crunch through leaves in autumn, and he would hold her up and swing her through so that she could do it. He bought her pretty clothes and never minded if they got dirty.

Then at 13 she went back into hospital for a major operation to correct the curvature of the spine. She was one of the first children in the area to have this spinal fusion. Jim remembers seeing her after the operation in plaster from her hips to her chin. She lay on her back in bed for months, as she had with the acute polio a few years before. When she finally came home she had to wear a large spinal brace. She remembers once being told off for scraping the wallpaper with it as she struggled upstairs.

The operation was a success and she was able to walk short distances without a calliper. At least she could walk and work. She was naturally short of stature, and her illness made her shorter. Her remarkable character may have been a result of her illness. But her most beautiful features were not: they were independent of experience – given as though to balance and to mock her polio-weakened body.[2]

Her years of illness must have had their effect on her personality, but for those around her it was difficult to judge. She was obviously determined, and determined in particular to succeed to the limits of her physical capacity. What she never would do was waste time. She had lost enough of it in Alton. But that didn't mean she was severe or dour. She took an innocent delight in doing the simple tasks. Baking cakes or going out were major events for her and she got a big kick out of them. Somewhere along the line she had known despair and bitterness. But the grieving was over and she was determined to get on with life, and get on with it on her own two feet.

This made for slight difficulties at home. Try as they might to develop their relationship, half a childhood away had loosened the family ties. Mavis had to break her parents' protective shell; watching their dear, wasted, defiant daughter taking on the world wasn't easy for them.

Once back at school she concentrated on typing because it would give her a career. She used to spend time in lessons wondering how she would manage to get to the next lesson. One teacher threatened her with a special school for children 'like her'. Fortunately she was bright and learnt quickly. She would have gone far, if she had been able to go far.

At 16 she left school and immediately took a typist's job locally at a haulage contractors. They sent a van each day to pick her up as she couldn't get on and off a bus. She could just use both hands to type but could only walk a few yards. As with Ian, an important advance came when she learnt to drive, and she passed her driving test first time; the only adaptation was an indicator, as she couldn't move her arm out the window. She could now decide on her own when and where to go out. Mobility and independence were hers at last.

She tasted life; she had boy-friends; she went off on holiday with girls in caravans. She managed the everyday things which most people would have thought were permanently beyond her. Whatever she did she delighted in; life was too precious to squander without savouring it. She was a bridesmaid at Jim's wedding, walking up the aisle on the best man's arm.

After a few years she met a young man and they decided to marry. They lived at first in a ground-floor flat and then moved into a bungalow. Mavis was working and keeping a house like anyone else. Then she discovered that everything, alas, was not as it seemed. She found that her husband was involved in homosexual activities, and soon he left her to live with another man. She was devastated. She had to go through an awkward and painful divorce and rearrange her life on her own. The local disabled group was part of the process. On that first visit she offered to be its secretary. She also met Ian.

*

Ian was bowled over by her. After the meeting they stood outside chatting long after everyone else had gone. Mavis invited him over to her bungalow for a cup of tea and a chat any evening he was free. Any evening he was free! Was she kidding? He hadn't had anything but free evenings since leaving Jersey. The next day he phoned her and they agreed to meet the next evening.

'I just couldn't believe it, I was so excited by the idea. I was like a schoolboy on his first date. I was like the proverbial dog with two tails. I went around with a grin from ear to ear. Then panic. What should

I wear? What should we talk about? I started to think about all the silly things that could go wrong, like spilling my drink and tripping up. Was it really a good idea? Sure, she was attractive and charming, but who was I kidding? Obviously nothing serious would happen. Since when were women like that interested in men like me?'

When he arrived at Mavis's they just sat and talked. He felt entirely natural in her company. He hadn't felt so natural in anyone's company since being disabled. Both of them seemed to be able to open up and talk freely without any worries about offending or shocking one another.

Though they were comparative strangers, they talked of things they had hardly confided in anyone. Ian told her about his fears, anxieties and hang ups, about many things he had thought of before but had no one to tell. Mavis did the same. What impressed him was her lack of bitterness. He just couldn't believe that after all she had been through she retained such enthusiasm and spirit, and that she could relate it all with such humour. What he didn't see was that it was he who was giving her some of the reassurance and confidence she had lost after her divorce.

They ended their first meeting in the early hours with a kiss on the cheek. He knew that, if nothing else, he had found a friend he could trust.

*

Ian tried not to develop the situation into more than a friendship. He felt there was little he could offer to someone so capable and controlled. Their relationship would only ever be platonic. But he could not stop daydreaming. He was completely captivated.

The group had organised a visit to a riding stable which specialised in disabled pupils. Rather than go with the others, Mavis and Ian made their own way. They found somewhere for lunch. Ian was uncomfortable about not being able to fulfil the usual male role and carry the drinks from the bar. Mavis just laughed at him and did it herself. They chatted about it. What did it matter anyway? They were together in a pub enjoying their lunch. Who needed this stuff about role-playing? Ian began to relax and unwind.

They arrived at the stables a bit late. Mavis had already had a few riding lessons, and when she was offered a go on one of the horses she accepted immediately. It was nearly a disaster, because the handler ran off at a trot and almost unseated her. When she dismounted she was convulsed with laughter. Ian decided not to have a go. He didn't fancy ending up in hospital again, especially now. On the journey back Mavis offered to take him out in his car to give him some more experience. He agreed with little hesitation. It gave him an excuse to continue to see her.

'I hadn't expected to find anyone. I wasn't even looking. But here was someone I felt so happy and so comfortable with. Since meeting her my mind was on nothing else and I thought only of when we could see one another again. I was besotted and I was falling in love.'

They met frequently over the next few weeks, mainly in the evening, when they would go out for a drink and a drive. At the weekend they would spend their days driving around the forest, exploring the lanes and sometimes stopping for picnics. They were so happy Ian felt he was coming alive again. In the few short weeks he had known her she had opened his eyes to a whole new perspective. He had thought that much of life would pass him by and had slowly prepared himself to accept it. But, as Mavis pointed out, becoming independent was all well and good: it was the use of that independence to enjoy life that was important. He soon realised that he had only travelled half way down that path by going back to work. It was Mavis who showed him the whole way forward. For her part she had found someone who was devoid of the deceit she had so recently been exposed to, and who gave her understanding and a chance to share in life's opportunities once more.

Neurologically it was almost an attraction of opposites. Mavis could move one side but not the other, because the nerve cells in the spinal cord had been destroyed. She knew what to do but couldn't carry it out because she had no motor nerve cells to her muscles. Her sensation was normal, but the polio virus's infection had stopped movement of one side at the age of two. Ian, on the other hand, had normal motor nerves but a total lack of sensory cells to guide movement. He needed continuous thought and vision as a substitute. If love is the desire and pursuit of the whole, these two may have had an almost intuitive understanding of one another's difficulties.[3]

One evening they met at Mavis's bungalow and she cooked dinner. They chatted into the small hours and this time Ian didn't go home.

Except for his association with Lizzie he hadn't had a serious relationship with a woman since leaving Jersey, and he was terrified about how the situation would develop. Though he had gone over the scenario in his mind many times, he had never really pursued the thought seriously. His occasional difficulties in performance with Lizzie had not seemed to matter, but this was very different. He had no desire to humiliate himself or Mavis. More important, he didn't want to offend or compromise her. For her part Mavis too was apprehensive about how things were going. They talked over their worries and agreed that if they were going to start a serious relationship neither of them could think of anyone they would rather be with.

The following morning they were still friends and neither was unhappy about what had happened.

*

Over the next few weeks they saw more and more of each other and less and less of the disabled group. One evening after a drive along the seafront they parked the car at the top of Hillhead and watched the tide ebb away. It had been yet another hot day, and it was a delight just to sit in the cool breeze. It had been six weeks since they met. Ian couldn't believe how much his life had changed in so short a time. He knew he wanted to spend the rest of his life with Mavis. While he realised that there would be many problems, he was certain that together they would overcome them. He turned to her and asked her to marry him, and she said yes. As they hugged, Ian felt the tears streaming down his face. He had never been so happy.

Jim remembers meeting Ian for a chat. As the prospective brother-in-law he was to give him the once-over. Not that he was worried. Her family had noticed a huge change in her over the last few months. They got on well and at first he didn't notice much physically wrong with Ian. Jim's and Mavis's parents' main concern was the speed of their plans to get married. Mavis was strongminded and impulsive. She wanted to get married soon – why waste time? Ian agreed. The family may have had a few misgivings about the speed of developments, but they were powerless.

Ian and Mavis were married at a local register office on 13

December 1976 with two close friends, Paul and Hazel, as witnesses. The wedding was arranged quite quickly because it was a date few people wanted.

They had decided on a quiet affair. But Ian's mother, one of Mavis's close friends and about twenty girls from Ian's office had all found out and turned up to wish them well. In the evening they went to see Mavis's parents, who hadn't been able to come. Later they saw Ian's, who had got together with the family and put on a surprise party.

The intimate connexion between our physical and emotional lives is reflected in their shared language. We feel for someone, we feel an object. We fall for someone, we take them 'to have and to hold'. There are many such consonances. Love is of course not confined in expression to physical closeness. Sight and language are all important, though few have eloquence enough to express in words what they can show with a gesture. But often we only really become close (literally and metaphorically) to those we love, and the importance of touch cannot be overestimated. As John Lennon wrote – with challenging directness, if not much subtlety – 'Love is feeling, feeling love, Love is touch, touch is love.' There is a parallel saying in France that 'L'amour est l'attouchement de deux peaux' (Love is the contact of two skins). For Ian, robbed of this contact, love had to have a different manifestation.

'It took a while to come to terms with the fact that because of my disability there was no response or pleasure for me in touching. However, I soon realised it didn't matter. You see it's not the tactile aspect that really matters. It's having someone there to hold and hug that counts. It may have meant that our relationship was less sensual, but it was no less loving. Perhaps it was more loving and honest as we hugged and held each other for deeper reasons. The whole thing took on a different meaning. Perhaps love itself took on a different meaning. Love was the whole being together.'

Having to be more distant with people than he would have liked, when he did let someone in the satisfaction was immensely greater.

*

Mavis's bungalow was not conveniently placed for them, so they found a maisonette midway between their two jobs. Mavis had left her secretarial job by this time and become a communications officer at a local police station.

Ian tried his hand at decorating, changing the bedroom from its previous deep orange to a more subtle cream. He had to stand on the bed to reach the top of the walls, but he couldn't stop bouncing around or get into a proper position to freeze his body enough to use the paintbrush. Eventually he laid an old door across the bed, which allowed more stability, and by bracing himself against the walls managed to finish the work in this strange but effective position. It took two days solid. When he saw the result in daylight for the first time he realised it would need another coat. The two families offered to help, but he looked on it as a challenge and finished it before it finished him.

Once they had done up the inside of their maisonette Ian started on his greater love, the garden. Unfortunately this was so small that there was only room for the washing line, a chair and somewhere to put the cars.

In fact neither of them was particularly happy in the maisonette despite its convenience. Ian wanted a proper garden. They would both have loved somewhere with some land round it. But even with both of them working they couldn't afford it. They settled on an old-fashioned bungalow in a suburb of the city. Mavis's parents thought it quite unsuitable. It needed a huge amount of work, inside and out, to get it up to scratch. It also needed some basic adaptations.

Then there was the matter of the drop. The house was perched on the side of a steep hill, and 15-20 feet from the back of the house was a sheer drop half way down the garden. It was difficult to see how either Mavis or Ian could ever negotiate it. Even Jim, who had always tried to see things from his sister's point of view, had strong reservations about the place. But, as before, a combination of Mavis's spirit and Ian's stubbornness carried them through.

They bought the bungalow and started to do it up. It was a big job: so big that they let others help. Before moving in Ian painted the ceilings with a brush tied on the end of a broom handle. Michelangelo he was not, and painting white on white made it difficult for him to get a visual fix to enable him to balance, so he fell over a few times. He often went home in the early hours tired, aching and spattered with paint. But he did it.

At the front of the house there was also a big drop from the road into the front garden. Ian somehow manhandled some large paving slabs and set them on end as a fence. Then behind them he constructed raised flower beds so that he and Mavis could do the gardening more easily. At the back he made a large patio, again out of paving slabs. Jim remembers going round to help, though he can't remember just how Ian managed to move these great slabs.

Ian cleared a lawn at the back and bought a second-hand power-driven mower. When they got it home Ian plugged it in while Mavis made a pot of tea. Ian shouted for her to switch on the power. The mower took him completely unawares, knocked him over and, being self-propelled, careered across the garden scything through a new bed of plants. It was just as it had been in Jersey. Mavis was hysterical with laughter. She chuckled away for days, and would remind him about it whenever he got too cocky. They took the mower back to the shop and replaced it with an electric-powered number that you pushed. It really was a lot less bother with a hover!

He also built a patio at the back. Jim helped, especially with the large paving stones. He remembers it as hard work, so what it was for Ian can only be imagined. But Mavis loved the sun, and the patio was a wonderful sun trap. It had a fine view across the city and, much closer, of a group of trees. They loved to watch the birds coming and going to their nests. Next came the chickens. Ian hacked out the undergrowth half way down the garden and built a hen house. Russell, Jim and Brenda's son, used to go round to collect the eggs.

Within a year or so they had made it into a really pleasant bungalow, confounding the fears of Mavis's parents and others. More than that, they had made their own home: one which had taken far more effort to create than usual and was therefore valued far more.

Mavis was the first person to visit Brenda in hospital after the birth of her daughter Louise. Brenda remembers thinking how fortunate she was to be a mother while Mavis would never be able to be one. Ian and Mavis had decided against having children, feeling that it would be unfair on them to have parents who couldn't play football with them or swing them around the garden.

Still, Mavis showed no disappointment. She and Ian set about doing up their new home. They did all the decorating and tiling themselves. They were both working full-time, but they managed to do home improvements in the evening. If Ian ever felt like a rest he would take one look at Mavis and forget it. She was his inspiration.

Though understanding with others, she could be hard on herself and so, by extension, on Ian. 'If I can do it you can do it.' And do it he did.

Louise loved to go round to see her aunt and uncle. Now, at 17, her memories are faded and patchy. What she remembers is her aunt's beautiful smile, as she sat on the verandah in the sun. Mavis loved to cook cakes and biscuits for her. As for the polio, Louise remembers only that her aunt could not walk properly: for instance, when they went shopping at Sainsburys they were allowed to park close to the shop entrance. She doesn't remember any oddity at all in Ian. Russell likewise remembers collecting the eggs, but not that there was anything wrong with Uncle Ian.

All this was achieved with the ruthlessness towards wasted time that Mavis had developed during her illness. Just as blind people have to be careful where they put things down, so that they can find them again, so Mavis was miserly about her use of time. She had to plan all her movements ahead because she didn't want to waste any of them. She continued to ignore sympathy and she was equally hard on Ian.

'I thought I was bloody-minded until I met Mavis. She would say, "You've just come from the bedroom." "Yes," I would say. "Then why didn't you bring the cups out?" '

Brenda remembers once hanging out washing on the line. She had forgotten some article and went inside to fetch it. Mavis was angry with her for not thinking ahead and for using up precious movements unnecessarily. Mavis planned everything every day, doing as much as she could with as little wasted effort as possible. This may make her sound severe. Not a bit of it. The famous smile was nearly always evident. On the whole she was hard on herself, like Ian, but great company for others. She even insisted that Ian sometimes invite his father round for meals. She was the one who kept these evenings flowing, and she got on well with Popsy, whom she called her father-in-law. Popsy loved it.

They settled into a normal, enjoyable, mundane, married life. It was a life of unremarkable richness, like that of millions of others. But for both of them it was more than they could ever have hoped for. Through long years in hospital Mavis had missed out on her early family life and had never really regained it. Ian's childhood had also had its problems. He too had spent not months, but years, in hospital. Now they were able to devote themselves to one another. Together they could do far more than each could have hoped to do alone.

9

In the Bleak Midwinter

One January, after they had been married for about six years, Mavis came to Brenda complaining that she felt unnaturally tired.

Brenda just said: 'Well, have a few days off, you'll be OK.'

But Mavis wasn't to be fobbed off. She was never to be fobbed off. 'No. Listen, I'm really exhausted. I can't work properly. I just don't know what I'm going to do.'

Soon afterwards they were invited round to a friend's for a meal. After the main course Mavis excused herself and disappeared into the bathroom. She was gone a while. Then she returned and apologised for ruining the evening. She would like to go home as she was feeling unwell.

In the car she explained that, though her period wasn't due, she had flooded and had severe abdominal cramps. But as she hadn't ever been very regular with her cycle she wasn't unduly worried. She went to bed with a hot-water bottle and agreed to see the doctor next day.

Neither of them slept very well that night, and in the half-light Ian could see that Mavis was drenched in sweat. She woke in the early hours. She seemed delirious, and she was trying to get out of bed. He went round to her side to help, and as he pulled the covers away he could see that she had suffered another heavy loss of blood. She was beside herself with pain, and there wasn't anything he could do to help. She writhed around in the bed but refused to let him call the doctor. In desperation he went out to fill her a hot-water bottle.

When he came back she was sitting on the edge of the bed, doubled over in pain and clutching her leg. All she wanted was to get to the loo. She had no energy, and in desperation Ian put an arm round her shoulders and somehow managed to pick her up and carry her next door to the bathroom. He sat down beside her, afraid to leave her.

After a while she rallied and Ian returned to the bedroom to change the sheets. He fetched her a towel and a hot flannel, and she seemed a little better. They went back to bed, but a couple of hours later the whole experience was repeated.

In the morning, after a cup of tea, she felt much better. She promised to make an appointment to see the doctor later that day. Ian went to work and rang her. He was annoyed to hear that the surgery had refused a home visit and insisted she visit them. Mavis, ever the diplomat, had said she was feeling much better and thought the fresh air might do her good.

Ian got home early that evening to find her upset and agitated. At the doctors she had asked for a few days off, but the doctor felt she was over-reacting. This was the first time she had ever asked for days off, and now when she did ask the answer was no. The doctor thought that all she had to do was pull herself together. He thought the events of the night before had just been a heavy period.

Both Ian and Mavis felt it was far more than that, and were convinced that in fact she had miscarried. The doctor said they should have kept what went down the loo as proof. Neither could believe his callousness.

Once at home Ian rang the surgery and said they were coming round.

They were shown into the waiting-room. Ian would have none of it. He insisted on waiting in one of the examination rooms, as he knew it would save Mavis's energy if she could lie on a bed.

As she lay there he noticed how tired and frail she looked. He also noticed, for the first time, how much weight she had lost since Christmas. He felt angry with himself that he hadn't noticed before and had done nothing sooner.

The senior doctor came in, walked over to Mavis, pulled down her eyelid and said, 'You're anaemic. Come back tomorrow, and see your own doctor for a course of tablets.' With that he turned to leave.

Ian could take no more. He grabbed the man's lapel and insisted, first, that the doctor must listen to the story and, secondly, that Mavis should have a blood test the next morning at the local hospital. For good measure, he mentioned a Community Health Council he knew where complaints were registered against doctors. Stonily, the doctor agreed.

Ian took the next day off and went with Mavis to the hospital. The samples were taken. The results would come to the surgery in a few days. They returned home convinced that Mavis had miscarried, an opinion reinforced by a friend who was a nurse and who had had a similar experience.

That afternoon the surgery telephoned. Mavis was to go to the local obstetrics and gynaecology hospital, where a bed had been booked for her for tests. The nurse was reassuring, saying it was just routine and she would be in only a few days. Mavis, who had undergone more than twenty operations, was very upset.

They arrived at reception and gave Mavis's name. The nurse announced that she couldn't be Mavis since the only person of that name they were expecting was arriving by ambulance. Once that had been sorted out they were shown into a single room. While Mavis changed, Ian chatted with the nurse. She told him that they had expected Mavis to be admitted as a stretcher case because she was so anaemic.

In the evening Mavis's parents visited with Ian. They were all delighted to see that she was looking a little better. Apparently she had been given a transfusion, and once again there was colour in her cheeks. The doctors planned some investigations for the next day. Meanwhile she was on bed rest. Her parents laughed about Ian having to fend for himself for a few days. As they parted, he promised not to burn the house down with his cooking.

Ian went home feeling better. At last Mavis was receiving the attention she needed. But he was still disappointed with himself for not having noticed her condition sooner.

The next day, when he visited her in the evening, he was glad to see that she was much more cheerful. The tests seemed to have gone all right and she thought she would be home soon. They laughed about how far it was from the car park to her room and how the long hospital corridors seemed to have been designed only for fit people.

He went home and slept rather better, but still not well.

The next day Mavis rang to ask him to pick her up. She had clearly been crying, and she explained that though she was allowed home for the weekend, she had to return the following week for an operation.

*

Ian phoned Brenda and asked her to come with him. Before they went in to see Mavis he was stopped by a nurse and taken to a young lady doctor. She sat down next to him and began to talk about Mavis, but without saying anything specific. Ian asked her outright whether they had found cancer. She said yes. Ian just sat there, saying nothing, and the doctor said nothing either. Ian asked if it was treatable. She explained that, though it was more advanced than they would have liked, they had every confidence in a good recovery. She sounded positive and encouraging. Ian asked how much Mavis knew. The doctor said she thought Mavis had guessed, though no one had actually discussed it with her. Ian asked the doctor to accompany him and tell Mavis exactly what she had just told him.

Since their first meeting, Ian and Mavis had never had any secrets. They had agreed that they would be totally honest with each other in any situation. They both understood only too well that it was the not knowing that was so destructive, and that they might be able to fight if they knew who and what the enemy was.

The doctor agreed. She gave them a couple of minutes together and then came into the room and explained the problem. Mavis lost her colour.

Brenda drove them home. Alone in the lounge they hugged and cried.

And when they had finished crying they talked. Mavis decided that the best thing was to play it down: to try to retain as much of a normal existence as possible. If the doctor could be optimistic, so could they. Her parents came round and they told them that the prognosis was optimistic. She broke down after they left. She felt so guilty for having let them down again; first there was the polio and now this. To make it worse, she had lost a close friend to cancer a few years before.

Mavis went back into the hospital for a hysterectomy. Unfortunately they found that the cancer had spread to her bladder and she wasn't allowed home to convalesce until it had recovered a little. She had recovered from the operation itself and couldn't understand why she was being held back. It was tough for Ian having to see her, and even tougher not telling her the reason. He felt terrible having to lie, after promising to be open and honest.

He was also having keep up an optimistic façade in front of the family. But he couldn't do it for long. One day he found himself able to confide in Brenda. They were sitting in the kitchen, and she was looking out of the window at the garden, when he said:

'They couldn't get it all out, you know, and the radiotherapy isn't going to do the trick either.'

Brenda had suspected the worst. At least by sharing it they were able to help Ian, as well as Mavis, cope as best they could. There were still laughs to be had, though. One of the other patients used to be visited by a man every afternoon. It was always plain to see that they thought a lot of each other. But then in the evening another chap would visit, but without the passion of the afternoon. His visits would end with a peck on the cheek instead of the blood-boiling throat-massage of the afternoon. Ian asked Mavis what the afternoon chap had that the evening one lacked. She replied that the evening man was her husband and the afternoon chap her local vicar, with whom she was having an affair.

*

When she was finally allowed home, Mavis spent her days sitting outside on the patio. She soon had a deep tan, and her hair, naturally blond anyway, was bleached white. It was uncanny, but she looked again as she had when Ian had first met her six years before: maybe with a little less weight, but very much the old Mavis.

It was the radiation treatment that really knocked her for six. She had two caesium implants, and she also made some outpatient visits to radiotherapy. She felt ill and low. Ian was by her side as much as possible, caring for her, always knowing the hopelessness as he watched her fight as she always fought, the cause already lost. She came through the treatment and went home looking even more drawn and gaunt. She could do little except sit out on her beloved patio.

Ian never gave up. He never stopped trying to make her life bearable: something she had shown him when they first met those few years before. He built her a ramp from the verandah down to the garden, ostensibly because they both thought at one stage that they might need a wheelchair. Mavis once confided to Brenda, 'I won't make old bones', but Ian just carried on. He continued to bed out plants in their garden though he knew Mavis wouldn't see them flower.

Like so many disabled people, Mavis had always lived at the peak of her abilities, working hard just to keep pace with everyday life. Running a home and doing a full-time job were extras. When her illness came along she had no reserves to fight with. As she got worse, the burden fell more and more upon Ian, both to nurse her and to cope with all the family and friends.

After a particularly bad day Mavis told Ian that she really felt the battle was lost. Rather than kid themselves any longer they should talk about how she wanted her life to be at the end.

At first Ian tried to talk her round to a more positive attitude, but they both knew she was right. She was terrified of dying, but one way of easing the inevitable, she said, was for her to die at home, in her own bed. With the help of the local district nurse and her own family they would be able to cope. She also said what she wanted to happen when she died; she didn't want anyone to see her then. She had given it all much thought. Ian was upset at first that she insisted on talking it all through, but then was grateful that she had the courage to talk so openly about her worries and fears and wishes. He realised that one of her main reasons for instructing him was to make it easier for him when the time came. For his part, he vowed to do everything she asked.

To her parents Mavis had always been the poor sick child who needed looking after. During their marriage Mavis and Ian had striven to escape from all that. Now that the nature of the illness became apparent, Mavis's parents were devastated and wanted to help care for her again. But Mavis wanted Ian, and Ian alone. For his part, Ian was committed to doing what Mavis wanted even if it meant crossing her parents. His protectiveness was a response to Mavis's request. Her parents were worried that she might not be able to get the care she required at home, while Ian was determined she should. No harsh words were exchanged, but Jim in particular could sense the strain.

*

They managed at home for several weeks with help from friends and a team of local nurses. Inevitably the pain got out of control and Mavis went to the local hospice for her regime of pain-killing drugs to be reorganised. She was frightened she would never come out again, and it was difficult to convince her that it was only a temporary stay. But the staff were superb and as good as their word. They treated her well, and as soon as the pain was under control she returned home.

Mavis knew she would change towards the end and she decided she would rather have people remember her as she was, when she was well, than as she would be at the end of a long illness. It fell to Ian, almost to Ian alone, to shield her from family and well-wishers. He was less than popular with many members of his family and close friends, but this was one wish of Mavis's that he could and would keep. A good friend of theirs helped out greatly at this time too.

Once Mavis came home again her new regime of painkillers worked well for a while, but as summer went into autumn the pain returned. One evening after a number of long days they realised that she would have to go back to hospital. As they talked about it, Ian was upset that her wish to die at home would not now be realised. Mavis kept her disappointment to herself. He was exhausted, frightened and bitter to see her dying so cruelly. Jim thought that he showed enormous strength and dignity in coping with the physical problems imposed on him by Mavis's illness. Despite the emotional vivisection he was suffering he presented an outward appearance of normality, as he had promised Mavis that he would.

She was admitted next day. Ian stayed with her as much as possible. Over the next few days he sat holding her hand, chatting, laughing once or twice; but more often they cried. Ian desperately needed some support, and he phoned his mother, who was now living alone in Jersey. She flew over the next day. He took her to see Mavis and left the pair of them hugging each other and crying.

There were two chaplains attached to the unit, and one evening one of them stopped to speak to Ian, inviting him to join in his services. Ian exploded. How could a loving God do this to Mavis? If there was a God, Ian's thoughts towards Him at that moment were not benevolent. Singing carols in his praise was just not something he could do. The chaplain took all this in his stride. If he could do anything, let him know. Was there a special carol that the choir could sing for Mavis? Her favourite carol was 'In the Bleak Midwinter'. Later that evening, as he sat down with Mavis, the choir stood outside her door and sang the carol. It was the last song she heard.

By then it was obvious that time – the precious time she would never waste – was running away from her. She rallied, became brighter and more peaceful, and then deteriorated once more.

Jim remembers one Sunday evening when he, Ian and a friend were all sitting with her. Her breathing got worse and they gave her an injection, which eased things considerably. Just after midnight Jim left, unsure of what more he could do, and with the prospect of a busy Monday ahead.

She died peacefully that night. Ian sat on her bed holding her hand, saying goodbye. When he walked away there ended the most beautiful chapter in his life. He stood in the corridor, never having felt so lonely or desolate. At five next morning he knocked on Jim and Brenda's door at home. They all knew why. Even Louise, who was 10, remembers waking up in the middle of the night when there was a knock on the door and knowing that her aunt had died. She died on December 6th and was buried on the 13th, their wedding anniversary.

*

Ian was determined to make all the funeral arrangements, partly for Mavis, but partly because he felt they might help him through. Before the funeral everyone gathered in their house. He sat alone in the bedroom remembering how, at a cremation service a year or so before, Mavis and he joked about the ease of access. They had laughed at how much more convenient a cremation would be for them since they wouldn't have to clamber over mud and grass to the graveside.

The chapel was packed, and Ian was grateful for once that he had an excuse to stare at his feet. He knew he would crumble if he caught someone's eye. The chaplain made the ceremony as positive as he could. When it was over, Felice said she was surprised that Ian hadn't cried. But of course he couldn't have cried, because tears would have distorted his vision: he would have lost his balance and fallen over. Even on this day the dreadful neuropathy would not allow him to show his feelings. He had spent hours crying with Mavis and knew that he would spend many more hours crying for her. But on this day he couldn't. For the rest of Christmas Ian avoided seeing people, though they were generous in their offers of help and support. Felice stayed with him, and they had a few quiet weeks. She returned to

Jersey in the New Year.

Once she had left he started to look for somewhere else to live, as he couldn't endure being alone in the bungalow. He bought a flat – an anonymous flat – in the centre of the city. There was no garden, there were no chickens, there was no patio. He did a bit of decorating, managing to put the wallpaper on upside down. But his heart wasn't in it, for there was no Mavis. For months he just existed, and then slowly he tried to pick up the pieces. The only way he could, he found, was to spend time alone. Apart from work he saw few people. He started going to the forest more often to observe the animals and take photographs. His life reverted to the struggle for existence it had been in the early days. And all the time he discussed their time together he only ever mentioned once the fact that she had polio.

10

Life's Work

Ian entered the Civil Service at the lowest level as a Clerical Assistant. His first job involved checking and completing documents before they were computerised for statistical analysis. It was as deadly as it sounds but, with the people around him and the concentration required, he found himself fully occupied.

He was taken on in the same capacity as an able-bodied person, and that is how he conducted himself. He began by using two walking sticks, but on finding he could manage without he soon left them in the car. He would turn down offers to step into a full lift at lunchtime, or at the end of the day, for fear of an accident. He preferred to have a shortened lunchbreak or be late home rather than risk an awkward situation. But on the whole he fitted in well. If he had thought allowances were being made over and above what was absolutely necessary, he would have left.

He approached work as an able-bodied person, and his bosses and fellow-workers considered him one too. He was sometimes asked if he would like any of the aids available to disabled people, but he always turned them down. The only concession anyone remembers is the offer to get him a drink or a snack from the passing trolley so that he wouldn't have to get up.

However, to say that he was never treated differently from anyone else is a slight exaggeration, if only because he managed to combine a consideration for others with a truly warped sense of humour. Perhaps that is why he got on so well with John Westland, his immediate superior, who was similarly twisted. Once he had mastered the work, his high spirits showed themselves. If colleagues went to a pub for lunch on a Friday, he would soon become the centre of attention, cracking jokes and generally making everyone laugh.

Soon after he began work his desire to appear unaffected by his condition was nearly his undoing. A pretty girl he hadn't noticed around the office once asked, in passing, if there was anything she could get him from the drinks machine. He said he would love a cup of tea and she brought it. They got to chatting and eventually she asked if he was ever going to drink the tea. He had been leaving it, as usual, until it was cool. He had the choice of explaining why or risking tea down his trousers: honesty or pride? Naturally he chose pride and just about managed to drink the tea without disaster. That night he practised picking up these cups until he was satisfied he could do it.

John never asked Ian about his disability and Ian never volunteered anything. John soon realised that he would have told him if he had he wanted to. Of course people had realised something was wrong when Ian joined the office, and they used to ask about it. He usually gave an evasive answer, which was like saying, 'Let's not go into it', so most people didn't.

Ian's sense of humour did not stop short at his boss. Once he arranged for John to have a pre-recorded phone call from Santa Claus. For a full twenty seconds John assumed it was a live caller and conducted an animated conversation. It was only with the question 'And have you been a good boy this year?' that he realised he had been set up. By this time everyone in the office was hysterical.

Ian recognised instinctively who was gullible and teased them mercilessly. The stuffy had the rise taken out of them too. One chap who enjoyed a joke but had no ability to laugh at himself seemed the perfect target. A coupon requesting information about catering equipment was sent out in his name. Two sales reps escorted by a security guard turned up at his desk to interview him. He wasn't amused.

Oddly, though these pranks might have backfired, with Ian they didn't. In the office no one had a bad word to say of him. He always had time for any problems. He would slide a little joke into a conversation, lightening the talk without trivialising it.

*

Ian had to function in a world which gave few concessions. The office was quite a hostile place for him. For instance, walking round could be hazardous. Some of the floors were highly polished or had loose carpets. He always had to anticipate trouble, and if he saw a shiny floor[1] he would tense up, and the tenseness often gave him a backache. At corners he would go wide and slow. Once he might have enjoyed bumping into a young secretary, but now he would just be sent sprawling. He had to be careful of any disruption of his posture.

Once someone came up behind him and gave him a congratulatory pat on the back. He all but collapsed. Without any postural reflexes, standing up required continuous thought. He couldn't adapt to rapid changes imposed from outside. Once his posture had been altered in a way he couldn't predict visually he lost his map of where he was and risked falling.[2]

When we fall normally we put our arms out, or brace ourselves, or decide to relax. Even falling is done with direction and purpose. Ian, however, had none of this control and so was more likely, not only to injure himself, but to land in an awkward position. At Odstock much time was spent trying to teach him the least harmful, most relaxed, way to fall. Such falls not only were painful but exposed his lack of normality to others. It was not only his pride that was hurt. The fragility of his recovery was revealed.

He learnt quite quickly to carry papers round the office. Into his hand they would go; he would make a grip and keep it as he set off. At the end of the journey he often noticed they were creased. Or his hand and arm would begin to feel tired. He would look down and remember why. When walking he would concentrate only on his progress and forget he was holding papers. To keep them from falling he would increase the strength of his grip, to be on the safe side (and partly so that he could gain feedback using a sensation of muscular tiredness). The papers would be sweaty and crumpled and his hand exhausted. He soon arranged to put them in a folder if he had to take them round the office.

He wasn't always in a position to control or predict what happened. For instance, one day he met John in the car park. 'Please Ian, could you take these papers up to the office?' He thrust them into Ian's hands and walked off.

Ian began to fumble. Had he got his hand through the bag handle or not? Had he got all the papers? It all happened too quickly for him to assimilate. He had to stand there calmly trying to arrange papers, fingers and hands into a manageable form, as if trying to undo a difficult knot.

Rarely did he give in. One area of difficulty that persisted was his writing, which was slow and never clear. At one stage he was asked to write the minutes of some meetings. He accepted reluctantly. He found it extraordinarily difficult both to listen and to write and, of course, to sit. He couldn't take in what was said and also write. Fortunately they had back-up minutes made, and after four or five times he was relieved of the duty. But this was the only part of the work he didn't master. Much of it involved personal computers. Though he was slow, he found it easier to use a keyboard than to write. He hated to give in to his disability and focus attention on it, but on this occasion he had little choice.

He learnt to negotiate the ramps and slopes he met around the office, and to manage stairs. Nothing, however, was ever relegated to the reflex, the unthinking.

'I was walking down a slope at work, one that I don't normally use. As I approached it and before I even stepped on it I had planned how it would be tackled. I assessed the surface and the angle of the slope, inclined my body in sympathy with it, shortened and slowed my pace and widened my stance. All this I did while I was discussing a technical problem with a colleague. I have to be aware of every situation before I go into it.'

Stairs and slopes were visible; but high-rise office buildings create high winds, and high winds cannot be seen. Such winds altered his postural relation to the visual horizon in unpredictable, unfelt and constantly changing ways. He therefore tried to avoid gusty days and places. If he had to face such a situation his posture became stiffer, his legs straddled apart, and his concentration increased.

At work the social rules were fairly well established. Secretaries and executive officers all knew how to behave and how far they could play around. Once he had got to know them he would occasionally go out with friends after work. But while they unwound he soon found that he couldn't relax. If anything, his vigilance and uncertainty increased, because they would go to places with difficult terrain for him. People were far more likely to bump into him. Pubs were often dimly lit. He had to learn to appear to be enjoying himself in such places. He hated any act he was forced into; he hated not being able to let himself go. In one pub the only seats were barrel tops. He tried one, but the position was so difficult that he had to leave straight away. Such places were a nightmare.

'I always have to take everything in before I do anything. Where I will sit depends on whether or not people can come up behind me, and whether I have to make a silly movement to get in and out of the chair. I have to consider many things you take for granted. Your reflexes will get you out of new situations, but I have to try to anticipate. In a dimly lit restaurant, there may be a dark or patterned carpet with a hidden step. That can be a catastrophe, because once I've tripped I usually fall.'

*

It annoyed him that he needed more personal space than others, and had to have an area around him he could control and feel safe in. When he went back to visit friends in Jersey they automatically greeted him in the French way with a kiss on both cheeks. This posed problems because for a moment he lost visual contact with his feet and body. He wouldn't decline the gesture and admit his disability. He had to concentrate especially hard until the greetings were over and he was once more in control of his body space.

He dreaded the first office party. It was held above a pub, and he had to wait until everybody had gone upstairs before giving himself an uninterrupted climb. Unfortunately a group of latecomers arrived as he was half-way up and pushed passed him. Ian had to freeze as best he could to avoid falling. When he got upstairs the room was dark and crowded as he had expected. He headed for the first chair he could find and sat down. Unfortunately, when everyone else sat down for the meal, he found he was sitting at the top table. John looked at him none too happily, but there wasn't anything to be done about it. Ian hated drawing attention to himself, but sometimes it was unavoidable.

Public loos[3] were other places that specialised in subdued lighting, and sometimes he had difficulty locating the zip of his flies. Someone suggested a dab of luminous paint, but all agreed that that was going a little too far. Anyway, it wasn't just the zip which proved difficult to locate.

An enduring problem was that everything had to be planned. If he went to a restaurant he had to choose one without steps up to it. He had to be able to park the car fairly near, preferably not in a multi-storey car park. He would always choose a restaurant which wasn't too busy and meals which were easy to eat. Fish was out because of the bones, spaghetti because it was too messy. He opted for an endless diet of stews which could be eaten with a fork. He has often not eaten because the effort in movement was too much for him.

He only met one person who was antagonistic to him because of the disability. This was a temporary boss who complained about Ian's writing. It came up at a job appraisal. By now he was quite able to defend himself. Had anyone ever had a problem reading his writing? Had wrong information been gained because of his writing? To both questions the answer was no, and it was the boss's standing that fell.

He did have a slight battle over parking, however. It was very windy around the big office block and he sometimes found it difficult to walk even fifty metres from his car. One disabled girl was blown over twice. So he went to the Personnel Officer to ask for a parking space nearer the door. It couldn't be done, she said, because all those slots were for high-ranking officers. Ian left it, because it was summer anyway. But by winter he found that the problem was just as bad. So he went back, only to receive the same answer. This time he went on about recent government legislation which decreed that all disabled people had to have access to parking as near as possible to the point of entry to their place of work. He had made up the dates and acts but it sounded feasible and he knew it was based loosely on fact. It did the trick and some sensible spaces were allocated a few weeks later.

In fact more good came of it. Another Personnel Officer heard of it and consulted him about how the office environment and its safety could be improved. She was astonished when he described his entire floor, recalling every loose joint of flooring, all the bubbles in the fitted carpets, the slippery ramp, the trailing wires, the heavy doors and a dangerous step. He knew the contours of his floor like a map, since in order to get around he had to negotiate all these potential hazards which, to most other people, were invisible. To her credit, she took his advice and did what she could.

As Ian says, in asking for a few extra things disabled people are not being difficult or demanding. They are just trying to have their life made a little easier so that they can be on an equal footing with others. Often the simple things which make their life easier also help the able-bodied.

Though he had gone into the Civil Service at its lowest grade, he was determined to make a success of it. Eventually he went before the Promotions Board. He gave one of the best accounts of himself of anyone in the office and was promoted. He soon moved on to the coding and processing of data on congenital malformations. This was regarded as among the most important work undertaken, whose usefulness, in an ocean of statistics, was for once readily apparent. John remembers Ian's work in this field as of the highest quality both in efficiency and care. Perhaps the experience of his own illness focused his attention. He was in the team on merit. He wasn't being carried for his disability, but needed for his ability.

He settled in and over the next few years began to enjoy the responsibility of his work and the team-work of which he was part. He told only a few people of Mavis's illness, but he had long periods of leave and the word filtered round. Though John knew, it was tacitly agreed that he wouldn't fuss. When Ian was able to be at work at this time everyone carried on as normal, for which he was grateful. He was surprised and moved when so many of them came to Mavis's funeral.

*

After Mavis's death work assumed a greater importance. It occupied his time and forced him into the company of others. For a while his life revolved round his work. Outside he did the household chores and occupied his time, but it was at work that he could escape from the memory. His life became his work. For their part, his colleagues did all they could to help, which was to show him that life continued. He might have tried to throw himself completely into work, but of course his condition never let him forget it and prevented him from total absorption in anything.

One of his jobs was to liaise with the computer division which organised the processing of data. This was an integral part of his job and he had been doing it for years before Mavis's illness. One of the staff was a girl called Linda, who had joined two years before. Though she had had many long phone calls with him she had never met him and knew little except that he took his work seriously and had a wicked sense of humour. Once, when he sprained his ankle, she called him 'Hoppity'. It was only then that someone told her he was disabled. She felt terrible. She asked around the office but no one could tell her much about the disability. Nobody had ever been told much.

When he came back after that Christmas they started their phone calls again, and again he came over as being both good at his work and fun. She discovered his birthday was in May and made him a cake. They met properly for the first time when she arrived with a coconut and lemon gateau.

Over the next few months they saw each other quite often and got on well. She sent him some photographs of the Royal Wedding and as usual he couldn't resist a prank. Knowing of her phobia he sent them back with a plastic spider in the envelope. He wasn't really ready for another relationship, however. He was wary of being hurt if things didn't work out. He thought maybe he was letting Mavis down. Poor Linda was frozen out.

The trouble was that he couldn't find the words to tell her why. She was puzzled where she could have gone wrong and not a little hurt. Fortunately she hadn't told the people in her part of the office about their friendship, which made the end easier, but there were still embarrassing moments when they saw each other in the corridor or at lunch. For a good eighteen months he couldn't bring himself to talk to her. He felt guilty over the way he had treated her, but couldn't, at that time, bring himself to act in any other way.

A few months after Mavis's death he transferred from congenital malformations to the department's computer division. He felt that a change in topic would absorb him enough to soften the events of the previous year. It didn't, and though he was working with a good team he couldn't settle. He tried for a while, but computing was less enjoyable and less immediately interesting. So when John had a new package to pursue on hospital statistics, and knowing that Ian was unhappy, he arranged through an understanding Personnel Officer for him to be transferred.

*

At this time he was desperately unhappy in his work and in his home life, such as it was. He began to neglect himself, and consequently developed bad backache. As he was a tall man, and stood by bracing the back as best he could without feedback, back trouble wasn't surprising. It came and went, but he had to be more and more careful.

Once, however, he put his back out severely and, as luck would have it, had a bout of flu at the same time. One he might have been able to ignore, but the two together incapacitated him totally. He retired to bed and telephoned his mother to come over from Jersey to stay with him a few days. Living on his own in a small flat he just couldn't cope. Felice came to look after him just as she had at the start of his illness. He was almost as helpless as he had been originally.

For several weeks he was bed-bound. Some of his relations wondered if everything had become too much for him. He was certainly low. But he hung in there, as he always had. An X-ray at the local hospital showed that there wasn't anything seriously the matter with his back, though because of his posture the normal curvature of his spine was deranged. He was told that things ought to improve in time.

His absence from the office worried his colleagues. John went round to visit him and was shocked to see just how low he was. At work they put a cardboard box out for people to drop things in for him; soon it was full of biscuits, cakes and canned foods. Then word got round that he had the flu, and soon there were several boxes full. When they went to see him they had a car full. They filed in to visit him, complete with a Christmas tree covered with fairy lights. He was overwhelmed by their kindness, and it did much to cheer him up. Slowly the flu got better, and with bed rest his backache improved.

John and Ian worked together again for several years before Ian went before another Promotion Board. He acquitted himself pretty well. In fact one of the outside panel members confided in John that Ian had given one of the best interviews he could remember. He was given the title of Executive Officer.

*

Even after several years the office building could still prove dangerous. Ian had always avoided the dark, but at times he had to rely on electric light. He had learnt to use stairs, but it was a slow process and consumed his concentration and mental energy. So he often took the lift. This was a difficult place too, even with the lights on, since the visual horizon gave no clues to the up/down motion. Ian's technique was to find a corner, lean into it and brace himself.

One day the inevitable happened: the lights in the lift failed when Ian was alone in it. In a split-second he had to decide whether to fall into an unknown posture and risk hurting himself, or brace himself and try to remain upright. He chose to stand and consciously stiffened all the muscles of his back, legs and arms to maintain the posture. Fortunately the lights went back on again in a few minutes. But even after so short a time he was physically exhausted, covered in a cold sweat and utterly drained of his precious mental energy. A man not given to exaggeration, he said it took him several days to recover, something unimaginable for an able-bodied person. He ached all over from the physical strain. More important, he took several days off, resting his mental concentration, before he felt able to engage in the effort of daily living again. John remembers the incident well. Someone reported that Ian was stuck in the lift without lights. The rescue party proceeded with little sense of urgency. Once they had got him out he looked a bit tired, but no one thought much more of it. No one had any idea how serious the situation had been, or how mentally exhausted he felt.

*

After Mavis's death everyone at work had been very kind, and they helped him greatly during the week. But outside office hours and at weekends he was more at a loss. Home was solitary, and he turned to the natural world for time and space to heal himself. In the forest and on the foreshore, inhospitable places for him with their uneven ground, fallen trees and slippery banks, he would go armed with binoculars and camera. He would meet fellow naturalists to exchange information about the location of animals and rare plants, but it was through the company of creatures and plants that he regained some balance and perspective.

He would get up at unearthly hours to watch birds at a nearby estuary. Though he wrapped up in warm clothes, there were still problems. Once, for instance, he was following a flock of birds as they took off. All was well until he had to stare into the wind. Then the cold air made his eyes water and he was unable to maintain his stance. He even had to be careful watching a flock of birds at dawn on a lonely foreshore.

The forest remained his special place and he would spend hours watching animals from the trees.[4] Deer were his favourites. Sometimes he would visit the haunt of a family often enough and quietly enough to be tolerated by them at a distance. Then he could observe them, at rest, or with their young, or feeding or rutting. It is difficult to think of more difficult terrain for him to have tackled, with uneven ground, branches overhead and twigs on the floor. The deer of course watched back. Once one came quite close up to him as he was standing still and regarded him, as if to say, 'What's wrong with you then?' He finds it hard enough explaining to a friend, let alone a deer!

At times in the forest he over-extended himself. He once tried a narrow bridge. The further he went, the less confident he felt. But as he couldn't turn round and could hardly jump into the stream, he had to go on, fully tensed up. By the time he reached the other side he was both mentally and physically exhausted. In marshy ground, if his boots began to be covered in water or mud, he had to take urgent action or risk a fall. On one occasion his feet were covered in mud and he had to wait, where he was, as still as possible, until he was helped out.

'I've accepted that long walks are out, so I plan what I want to see. I have, what many don't have, time to spare. I can't say, "I'm disabled, so I won't do things." Sometimes I've got to have a go. It's only by doing it that you'll know. For instance, I've gone walking on snow to get a good shot for a photo. I know it's stupid – I fell over, hurt myself and smashed the camera. I've done it a couple of times. I have to do it. Why do I still get angry when I fall? But, hell, if I do it – I get immense satisfaction from pushing myself and achieving something.'

He has some beautiful photographs of deer. In each case he remembers not only the scene, but also how difficult or easy it was to take the shot. Mostly he used a tripod, because he would start to wobble if he held a camera and looked at the world through a lens. Even a tripod was difficult, since the camera was at too awkward a height for him to see the shot. With a long lens the problems were literally magnified. Having to carry a camera and a tripod hardly made him the quickest naturalist in the world, and he would often plant himself in one spot and wait for the animals to come to him.

Ian's enjoyment of any kinetic melody – in a child, a puppy, a ballerina – may have been heightened by his illness. Rather than making him shun the beauty of movement, his experiences seem to have given him a finer and deeper appreciation of it. He has had to think about his movements far more intensely than any choreographer. His interest in such graceful animals as deer is hardly a coincidence.

Slowly he was coming to terms with things once more. He found a new flat nearer his work. It was further from the forest, but a much lighter and more optimistic place in a better neighbourhood. It was a sign that he was beginning to look forward once more.

Work gave Ian financial stability, which in turn enabled him to develop his hobbies of photography and nature-study. It allowed him his longed-for return to the real world. After Mavis's death it helped him by occupying his time and by showing him that life had to go on. For a while his life became his work. He met people who became good friends. Yet his old aversion to offices and large organisations was never completely lost. He dreamt of becoming his own boss again – as he would have been as a butcher; perhaps in a software company, or helping to run a tea-room or guest house for the disabled. The years went by. While he worked he was sustained by dreams.

11

The Physiology of Cheating

In the assessment of patients with neurological problems one technique is to give the subject – with, say, weakness after a stroke – a specific movement to perform and see whether he improves with time. Any improvement is assessed in terms of neurological recovery. Such an interpretation, however, is too simple. Training and repetition by themselves may improve performance. One way this factor may be eliminated is to begin the assessment only after the subject is familiar with the task.

But in many complex tasks subjects also learn alternative ways of performance. A simple example is the way Ian learnt to distinguish the shapes given to him by a physiotherapist at Odstock, not by active touch, but by sound. This is an obvious example and one that could have been discovered simply enough, though we should remember that the physiotherapists thought Ian's neuropathy must have improved, to explain his 'recovery', when in fact there had been no change in his neurology. In more complex tasks patients devise their own tricks to get round difficulties. At the end of a period of assessment they may have improved by 'cheating' within the context of the test.[1] It is often this very cheating that indicates what neurological function is possible and shows off the individual's inventiveness at its best. But often it is not focused on because it is not part of the main experiment.

There has been no neurological recovery in Ian's neuropathy below the neck since the day he went into Jersey Hospital. He was told at the time that he wouldn't walk again. How has he managed to 'cheat' on such a gigantic scale?

*

Ian started with two advantages, without which his recovery wouldn't have been possible. First, since the illness befell him at the age of 19 he had already laid down all his motor programs. He had unconscious memories of how to walk, dress etc. He is sure that if he had had the neuropathy as a baby, before acquiring these programs, he wouldn't have been able to recover.

That is one reason, it will be remembered, why he is sympathetic to those people with cerebral palsy who have been brain-injured at birth. They are disabled not only because their movement commands are incoherent or are ignored by the damaged nervous system, but also because they have no knowledge from experience of the correct commands to be made. One of Ian's problems with swimming, apart from the worry of being in the water and having no clear image of his body, was that he hadn't learnt to swim before. He had no idea what he had to do.

At a common-sense level it is easy to imagine that having these motor memories was a help to him. He knew how to walk, dress and feed himself, and his rehabilitation was aimed at helping him recover those memories. It is more difficult to explain exactly how they were useful, since these programs are not accessible to the conscious level at which he had to initiate all movement. Head's movement schema must have faded without constant refreshment. Ian simply says, again and again, that he knew what he had to do for a given movement and that it helped. He would think that he was once able to stand and then puzzle out how he could stand again, not with the same motor programs but with ideas of his own.

This may suggest that, once he has made a voluntary command to move a limb, some of the neural signal goes through a circuit which accesses part of the old involuntary motor programs at an unconscious level. Just as rainwater tends to run off a hill in established streams, so a neural command may be directed along the most used pathways, even without feedback. These pathways would tend to be the ones used before the neuropathy and established by the normal programs built up before the illness. The programs are established through conscious activity and consolidated at a lower level and thereafter remain involuntary. Ian is not sure whether these do still exist for him. He once described the nerves as being a memory net the use of which he no longer had the luxury of.

It should be stressed, however, that all his movements involve some conscious thought, and that all are abnormal. None of the movements in the repertoire he has built up could be mistaken for natural ones. If such channels do exist, at whatever level, and have aided his recovery, they have lead to movements unrecognisable when compared with those they produced before his illness. Each time he wants to write he has to find a new way; the paper and pen are different, the angle of his arm on the page has altered, he has to anchor his forearm differently, and so on.

Any movement also has a complexity in execution which is not always apparent. Consider a simple single movement to raise the arm. Let us assume that one muscle contracts to raise it and another to lower it. It should not be thought that when one muscle contracts the other relaxes completely:

> The relaxing muscle has not given up all effort but is controlled in its yielding, with as fine a sense of adjustment as is the action of the contracting muscles. Nothing appears more simple than raising the arm; yet in that simple act, not only are innumerable muscles put into activity, but as many are thrown out of action and under the same act of volition.[2]

Even simple movements require subtle co-activations of many muscles. This coordination is normally automatic and below consciousness. The relative loss of this stable unconscious use of the antagonistic muscle to refine even simple movements is one respect in which Ian's new voluntary movements differ from his previous ones. He has had to learn movements at their simplest irreducible level, and this has rendered them crude, in the sense of being graceless.

When performing a movement that normally involves several muscles simultaneously, Ian tends to use one muscle, the prime mover, to the relative neglect of the others. When performing a movement which necessarily involves activation of many different muscles he has to think ahead. For instance, if he wants to move an object he is holding from his side to the front of him, he first has to think that he must lean back a little to prevent the extra weight in front from pulling him over.

His stance and walk cannot be mistaken for that of a normally innervated man. He stands by excessive co-contraction of the back muscles and the muscles of the anterior thigh and hip. Since he has to maintain the stance by constantly contracting these muscles, the posture is much more tiring than a normal posture, in which standing is achieved by subtle balancing between various muscle groups, which contract small amounts infrequently.[3]

Seeing him walk, one's immediate impression is of slowness and deliberation. Though it is achieved with relative economy, it still gives his gait a ponderous, stilted quality. He relies on the hip and thigh muscles more than is normal, and on the muscles which move the ankle less. He has to put his feet down an abnormal distance apart for balance. To avoid scuffing them on the ground as he brings them forward during walking he turns them outwards at the knee and the hip. Another way of preventing the foot hitting the floor would be to elevate the hips. But he didn't chose this option because any elevation of the body during walking increases his instability.

The feet are slapped on the floor without any yielding to the ground.[4] He puts the whole foot down and takes it off without the usual elevation onto the ball of the foot just before take-off. He does not trust the ankles, so he braces the whole foot on the ground. Similarly he always braces and straightens his knees before weight bearing, adding to the stiffness of the walk. His walk resembles Dustin Hoffmann's in *The Graduate* after he donned the subaqua suit.

He has to see all movement he makes. Looking at him from the side, we realise immediately that one of his main adaptations is to lean the head forward and downward so that he can see his body and legs at all times. To compensate for this the arms are carried further back than normal.

Detailed study of his walking pattern[5] has shown that he may make small contractions of the muscles of the calf as the foot reaches and leaves the floor. From this observation it appears that some very crude involuntary gait program is used, since he would probably not be able to think to activate these muscles.

Ian agrees. When he first began to walk, all movements required thought and concentration. But over the years he has found that he has not needed to think so hard about walking, say, on flat ground. Some small part of walking may therefore have been taken over by a gait program not reliant on peripheral feedback. But, as he pointed out, this is never the case on rough ground. Whereas walking in the

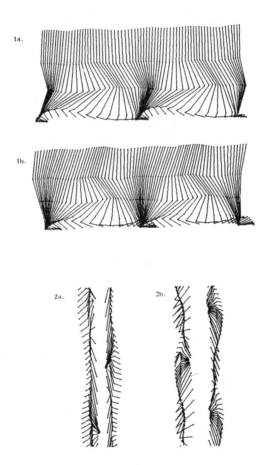

Figure 8. Gait analysis comparing Ian's walking with a control subject. The stick diagrams were obtained by attaching reflectors to Ian's shoulders, hips, knees, heels and toes and to those of a control, and recording and reconstructing from one side the pattern of their walk.

(1a) control, (1b) Ian, as they walk from left to right viewed from the side. Ian has to have his knee locked straight before and while his foot is on the ground. The foot is put down heel first, and his body leans forward during each step compared with the more upright body of the control subject

(2a) control, (2b) Ian, as they walk from top to bottom, viewed from above. Ian's feet are more widely spaced apart. The control's shoulders are always outside the hips, whereas in Ian his weight is more evenly distributed on each side of the weight-bearing foot.

able-bodied changes little from day-to-day, Ian finds that his ability to get around does fluctuate with his mood and health. On a bad day he has to think about all movement, and his walking then deteriorates.

Some aspects of walking are no longer dependent on continuous thought, but these parts are very small and have not allowed anything like a normal posture and gait. Nor have they allowed him the luxury of not having to think while walking.

Ian is ungainly but never clumsy. He can't afford to make any movement without extreme deliberation. In walking, as in other movements, the loss of proprioceptive feedback has robbed him of the involuntary control we take for granted. He has replaced it with a deliberation which, given the problem, can only impress us. Though his academic achievements were modest, the delicacy of his motor control reflects a lifetime's study of movement.

An earlier chapter described how primary sensations from the body are built up into far more complex sensory events before being presented to consciousness. A reverse process occurs in movements. We may decide on a movement and then that neural command is split involuntarily into the correct components for each muscle and distributed accordingly. In Ian we know that this split is simplified, but how he actually achieves it is unknown.

In the absence of feedback to guide and focus it the aim is not exact. With his eyes shut he can't move a finger on its own, since the ones either side make small movements too; and he sometimes has a mirror movement of the fingers of the opposite hand. The selectivity of movement commands appears to be dependent on peripheral feedback. The 'motor image' requires continual reinforcement or refreshment from the periphery.

*

The second function which helped his recovery was that he retained control of his head and neck muscles. The accurate postural control of the head, via the neck muscles, seems essential for the correct interpretation of signals from the inner ear organ of balance and for the eyes to give a stable view of the world. These two are dependent on reflexes involving the neck muscles. The neck muscles are also likely to be involved in postural adaptations of the body. It is doubtful whether these reflexes could have been replaced by voluntary movement, especially when the back of the neck cannot be seen.

Because of the problems with the mouth and pharynx I once asked him if he was able to sing after the neuropathy. He said, 'No, but I couldn't sing before.' The old jokes may be the best, but since making sound involves accurate exhalation, which in him depends on chest-wall musculature, some small defect cannot be excluded without experimentation. He has never noticed any problem with breathing.

Obviously the principal substitute for lost peripheral feedback is vision. For Ian and his body it is literally 'out of sight, out of mind'. But this visual substitution for the muscular sense should not be considered a simple matter.

There are some movements which seem to depend little on visual feedback for accuracy. When a child first walks and stands, she does not do so by looking attentively at her feet and body. No, she stands, looks ahead and feels for balance using the muscular sense. Whether running, hopping, skipping, or somersaulting, children are always on the move, learning movements not from visual inspection but from their muscular sense. A tight-rope walker proceeds not by looking at his feet, but by looking ahead, keeping his feet steady by this internal feedback. It would be no use to look at the feet, since the walker could never observe all the small movements of the ankles, let alone correct for them with visual feedback. A watchmaker, or an ophthalmic surgeon, may attend carefully to what he is doing, but he concentrates on the ends of the instruments, not on the muscles moving the fingers, which perform automatically.

Ian learnt again how to stand and then how to walk, dress, feed and write, all the time looking at the moving part of his body.

'How did I start? I knew I had to lift one leg, so I leant on the other. Often, while leaning, I would fall over, but gradually I learnt. I had to lean one way, but not too much, to give the other leg some leeway.'

The slowness, which is noticeable on flat ground, is magnified if the ground is not level. Ian has to approach uneven terrain as a climber approaches a pitch, working out the next move in relation to his present position and trying to predict the subsequent moves. Usually when walking or running over rough ground we don't look at our feet, but at the ground a few metres ahead. We assess the ground and then use an involuntary program and short-term memory to match our foot position and tension to where we will land. Ian always has to look at his feet since this predictive element is lacking, and he has to match footfall to terrain simultaneously. Not surprisingly he prefers even to uneven ground and grass to concrete. Grass is softer to fall on and less unyielding to walk on:

'If the world was a cricket pitch I'd be happy. If it was a pebble beach I might as well commit suicide.'

A severe limitation is that he has to have complete concentration on walking, or on any movement, so that he has no time for anything else. As at first sneezing meant potential catastrophe, now twenty years later he cannot daydream while walking. Sherrington wrote that in movement 'our minds are not concerned with the act, but with the aim'.[6] Ian has to be aware of both:

'I don't wander around looking for flowers. I look for paths. I just have to look at my feet. I lose peripheral things – the aesthetics do suffer. But I remember once being in London with an aunt who works in Covent Garden. We had a look round and a meal. I couldn't do much, partly because there were so many people and partly because I constantly had to stop to get my bearings. I had to plan my route very carefully. Then I stopped and thought, rather than just stop I'll stop and look around. I appreciated the view far more. I tell myself, and I think I can believe it, that when I am able to go down to the forest, I take in more than others, because I'm most aware of all the effort involved in my being there.'

Sometimes we become so interested in what is going on around us that we forget ourselves. However absorbing anything may be, Ian can never afford to be engrossed:

'I always have to think where I am and what I'm doing. I can never be completely absorbed. However beautiful the scene I have to concentrate on what I'm doing, especially on soft ground. Normally if I go anywhere I remember all the little potholes. You might remember a walk for the views. I just remember the walking.'

One of the greatest costs of his neuropathy is that it imposes on him a constant need to plan the easiest route. Like a chess player, he has to think several moves ahead. For example, each time someone comes into a room he has to see who it is, whether they will invade his body space, whether they will want him to do something, whether he will have to move to greet them or get out of their way. All the time he is out in a car or walking he is looking at the trees, or grass or litter, to see if there is a wind and to judge its direction.

But once, just once, he walked without thought:

'Have you ever gone somewhere and forgotten how you got there? Well, not long ago I was in the forest and for the first time since the neuropathy I actually made some steps, on a gravel path, without thinking about it. For a few seconds I couldn't remember.'

After fifteen years he had been able to use an unconscious motor program for a few seconds. If he had tripped he would certainly have fallen badly, since he had no idea where he and his arms and legs were. One object of learning these programs is so that we don't have to think of movements. It must take enormous mental discipline for Ian to concentrate continuously in this way.

The concentration is limited, both in the complexity of the tasks he will attempt and the length of time he can function. Sitting down in a stable position he does not have think much about his posture. He can then transfer an egg from one hand to the other. This is remarkable given the narrow scale of applied pressure between crushing the shell and dropping the egg. But he couldn't walk with an egg in his hand. Then the focus of attention would have to be on walking and the egg would be crushed.

This limitation in focus means that he has to work out priorities. Avoiding the dark might be considered troublesome but not too difficult. All things in life, however, are relative. He was recently invited to a Guy Fawkes party in a back garden. Though it was night-time his eyes had adapted to the relative darkness and the bonfire and house lights gave him enough light to see the ground and himself. He was enjoying the evening until the fireworks began. The brilliant flashes of light momentarily reversed the dark adaptation of his eyes and blinded him for the darker surroundings. He began to falter on his feet and had to tense up. The only way he could continue to enjoy the party was by not looking at the fireworks.

*

Some postures and movements are still difficult for him. He avoids them if he possibly can. He declined a friend's suggestion of a skiing holiday. That he was asked at all is powerful evidence of how successfully he has returned to a 'normal' existence. Kneeling on all fours is difficult. At the doctor's recently, he was asked to lie on his back on a couch. The couch seemed narrow and high. He was anxious, since he could see neither his body nor what he was lying on, and could have made little attempt at avoiding being hurt if he had fallen.

Talking to Ian it becomes apparent that his success has come from learning a limited repertoire of movements rather than the almost infinitely adaptable range we use normally. He sits, he stands, he walks. He tries to do these the same way each time. Even if he does not succeed he finds it easier to try to perform a limited number of movements. Familiar movements still require concentration, but they now need less than a movement not frequently employed. He estimates that safe movements frequently attempted take about half the mental concentration infrequent movements take, but he stresses that concentration still has to be applied. He hasn't jumped up or down since the illness and doubts if he could. Nor has he hung from a branch by the hands. He has wondered whether he could do either. He thinks he could learn to hang from a branch, but has never tried. They are, after all, useless movements which would only consume mental energy to no purpose.

In the use of his hands this adoption of a repertoire of movements has lead to a strict division of labour within. He was strongly left-handed before the illness and this has increased since. Tasks we might normally be able to perform with either hand Ian has relearnt with only one. Because of the necessity of voluntary concentration in all movements, learning to do something with one hand makes it no easier to do with the other. In some experiments we have shown that Ian's brain has undergone reorganisation. One of the parts concerned with movement, the cerebral hemispheres, usually responds to watching fingers move symmetrically: an electrical wave may be recorded over the left hemisphere after movement of the right fingers and vice versa. In Ian this response is very unusual. It is seen in the right hemisphere following movement of *either* his left or right fingers; he has relearnt to move with the dominant right side of his brain being involved in the sensory processing of movement related information from *both* hands.[7]

*

Though he does not receive information from the skin or muscles of the body useful for normal movement, he does have intact nerves conducting some sensations. It will be remembered that the smaller sensory nerve fibres in his peripheral nerves were intact. Temperature sensation is normal for hot and cold, and it colours his perception. He describes people as having a warm handshake. He uses temperature as a clue to movement in some situations. In bed he knows when his leg moves because he feels it cooler in a new position. He knows whether, with his eyes shut, his arm is raised because he feels cold air under the armpit.

Comparing the sensation he feels of a pinprick on his body and on his face, we see that pain sensation from sharp pricks remains normal. Such sharp stimuli are, however, but a small part of what we mean by pain. A more frequent pain is a knock or bump. This deeper, duller pain Ian feels slightly differently. He describes it thus, remembering what he was like before the neuropathy:

'Have you ever knocked your shin or banged a finger on a cold day when your leg or hand is feeling cold? Then the pain is more intense, lasts longer and is more unpleasant than when you hit yourself when you are warm. Well, when I feel pain it is now always pain of that more unpleasant kind.'

In neurophysiological experiments on human volunteers it is possible to block all the large fibres in a nerve, temporarily, and so mimic Ian's problem.[8] In this situation the unpleasant pain is also felt, suggesting that in some way large and small nerve fibres interact with each other in the transmission of nerve signals which are subsequently interpreted as pain. A bang on the skin never excites only pain nerve endings, but also pressure and touch nerve endings. These latter receptors might help us to interpret the limits of the pain stimulus and set its boundaries. In their absence a pure painful stimulus loses its normal sensory context and there is then a longer-lasting and unpleasant stimulus.

The poorly defined sensation of deep touch also remains. For Ian to feel pressure on the hand I had to grip it as hard as I could. Banging down with a heel on the ground or knocking something moderately hard (but not abruptly enough to cause pain) produces sensory feedback from these receptors. In practical terms this modality of deep touch is rarely felt by him and of no use.

*

Lastly it will be remembered that the non-muscle spindle intramuscular receptors responding to pressure, fatigue and cramp are also still functioning, and these are probably of considerable use. When carrying something and clenching it hard, it is the feeling of fatigue in the muscle that alerts Ian to a problem. Similarly if he has to bend or crouch – to take a photograph, say – it is fatigue that he feels. We all have a sense of intramuscular fatigue, but Ian seems to have become more sensitive to it, as a way of perceiving that a given muscle has been worked hard. It must be extraordinary to feel tired without a proper sensation of the movement that made you tired.

There are several elements in the control of movement, concerned with whether an arm is moved or not and the resistance it moves against, whether this is the weight of the limb itself or the weight of an external object being carried, for instance. Often the weight of such an object can only be judged once the movement has begun. We have all picked up a kettle we thought was full only to discover that it is almost empty, and find that our movement is too fast. Movement involves not only changing the position of a limb in space, but matching the force and rate of the movement to the external load appropriately.

'I know if a briefcase is full or not when I pick it up.'

'How?'

'Good question. I just know. How do you know normally? By pressure in the arm. Perhaps I'm getting some of that. Perhaps I know that the movement I get is not quick enough for what I'm putting in. To pick up a suitcase I first look down to check my feet, grasp it and start to pull up, like anyone else, except that I don't bend my knees. Then, if it doesn't come up there must be something wrong. I check that I'm not falling over, and if I'm not it must be because the suitcase is too heavy.'

The first thing he has to check when an object fails to move towards him is that he hasn't moved towards it, in this case falling over. He has little knowledge of his own stability in the world. Then he has learnt that a certain mental energy in his command to move leads to movement at a certain speed. He can judge this directly by sight. If a movement made with this mental force is slower than expected, the limb must have met resistance; the briefcase is unexpectedly heavy.

This perception, which is normally made through the muscular senses, he has learnt to make consciously with visual feedback.

However, even with his eyes shut he can still, just, judge the heaviness of an object. The perception is only one-tenth as keen as in normal people, but it is still present. This perception of effort, rather than of movement or position, arises in one of two ways: either entirely within the central nervous system, or from his remaining sensory nerves. There is evidence that the small receptors in the muscles can respond to the changes in tension within a muscle as a result of its contraction. Evidence distinguishing these two theories is not conclusive, but there seems to be sufficient evidence that the origin of his perception of effort is located in the remaining sensory nerves from muscles.[9]

This awareness of effort and fatigue is useful to Ian in letting him know if he is putting excessive force into holding an object, or standing in a certain way. It is also important in alerting him to possible injury before the part is painful. It was Bell who realised that the function of the muscle sense is not only to guide movement but to protect the body from incorrect and potentially harmful movements. The sense of fatigue Ian feels may prevent more serious muscular sprain.

As with other patients who have lost peripheral feedback while retaining some motor power, Ian's limbs seemed at first to move on their own. Sometimes, sitting in bed, as we have seen, he would just turn away and the out-of-sight arm would fly up and hit him or his visitor. Gradually he learnt to subdue these movements. It was almost as important to prevent unwanted movements of one arm as to learn visually directed accurate movements of the other.[10]

When he is sitting down or standing against something, it is relatively easy. He wedges a hand or shoulder against something. Then he can detect a movement by a change in temperature or deep pressure and immediately look to see exactly what is going on. But he can also hold out his arm in space reasonably stably without looking at it. If an observer feels the arm, he realises that it isn't being held up by one muscle group, but that all muscle groups are tensed up against each other. It isn't surprising that Ian feels fatigue. With this technique he apparently gains feedback from the receptors of intramuscular tension. Such tensing may also occur in competition shots during target shooting, so that even in normal subjects the greatest stability may be achieved by bracing the arm. Ian can keep an arm relatively stable, but drifts still occur. He is aware of them but without vision does not know their direction and is unable to make corrections without looking.

This tensing of muscles to keep the arm or leg still has another purpose too. Nicholas Bernstein regarded motor learning, not simply as imposing the correct movement, but also as increasing the central nervous system's knowledge of the exact position of the limbs. The finer the control, the more important it is for the nervous system to know exactly where the arm is and the state of all its muscles in order to move accurately. A difficulty is that a limb may be in many different positions and have many joint angles. That is, it may have many degrees of freedom. Bernstein suggested that improvements in co-ordination are achieved by reducing to a minimum the degrees of freedom at the periphery. One way is to keep still:

> When someone who is a novice at a sport or at playing a musical instrument first attempts to master the new co-ordination, he is rigidly fixed...to reduce the kinematic degrees of freedom which he is required to hold. Invertebrate organisms have...mechanisms of muscular locking which eliminate such degrees of freedom which are unnecessary at any given moment...All lower forms of vertebrate possess analogous mechanisms. Lizards, snakes, parrots are as rigid as statues in the intervals between movements. Mammals find similar locking superfluous, and return to it only in cases of disease (e.g. in Parkinson's, catatonia, etc). In the norm there is no rest in mammals and human beings. Even the set immobility of a cat or tiger is quite unlike the immobile period in a reptile – it is sufficient to watch its tail.[11]

Thus one reason why Ian has become expert in keeping still is that it makes it easier for him to begin and then structure a movement. He agrees that freezing has such a use, but he always has to trade off the mental effort against the improvements it brings about. He can only do it for a short time, but it does allow him for instance to take a photograph bending down using a tripod. And there is no better freezing than in a photo.

*

If Ian has managed to learn to move again, what of his sense of body image, his sense of self, which we all have and which often persists even when a part of the body has gone? Patients who have had limbs removed often complain of phantoms. They feel the amputated limb, though they can see that it has gone. Lord Nelson wrote that he could still feel his severed arm, and he used this as evidence for the existence of an eternal soul. The phantom has a presence but can also be severely, even suicidally, painful.

Ian has a body image based on fatigue, temperature, deep touch and pain. Yet he considers his body image quite normal. Despite the absence of the perception of proper touch, movement and posture he has never felt the presence of a phantom; the remaining sensory modalities appear to have kept it at bay. But that is not to say that he hasn't had some abnormal sensations:

'If I think about it I tingle, not all over and not painfully, but it's there. Sometimes I don't think and it's absent, and sometimes I do and it's there. It's easily removed by distraction and seems worse in the hands.'

At first and only for a short time, he also felt dripping or spider-like sensations over his body.

The extent of his recovery is a moving testimony to his courage. But what has he not found a way to do?

Though he stands and sits he never adopts a good posture. Backache is a frequent, and occasionally a serious, consequence. The normal forward curvature of the base of the spine is absent. Unable to see his back, Ian walks with it braced as best he can, so that it is too tense and too straight. He has 'put his back out' a few times, with severe pain, so that he has had to go to bed for a week or two. Having comparatively little control over his movements, he is in a much poorer position to control his movement to protect the painful area. In his defence, however, 'bad backs' are common in his family, so it is probably not wise to blame the backache entirely on his neuropathy.

His focus of attention on movement is limited. Some complex tasks therefore present too many difficulties, or degrees of freedom, for him to attempt them. Intellectually demanding tasks, like taking minutes at a meeting, require too much of his attention for him to maintain posture. Likewise physically difficult tasks would take too much mental concentration. Some other apparently complex coordinations, like ironing while standing, he can do by keeping an eye on posture and concentrating on the task in hand.

He also comes unstuck when speed of movement is needed. He walks at a sedate slow pace, and he can't raise the pace at all – a great worry when he has to cross a road. There is a finite rate at which he can absorb the visual feedback involved in these movements, process it consciously and work out the command for the next move. No movement is ever fluent, since each has to be split into these components.

The enduring, profound and absolute loss is in active touch, in the apparently effortless manipulations and exploratory movements we make with our fingers and hands. Even using the closest visual inspection he can't use his hands normally, tending instead to employ his thumb and first two fingers in a pincer mode with the other two fingers tucked away. The intricate movements we make to grasp a cup, turn over the page a book, scratch our face or even pick our nose are gone, to be replaced by far slower and more ponderous movements.

Although some tasks have defeated him, he has recovered to a remarkable extent. His exploration of alternative strategies in movement and his maximising of the use of remaining sensations are a testament, not only to his persistence, but to his intelligence. The areas of movement in which he has not managed to 'cheat' his way into competence pale into insignificance when compared with what he has achieved. He has had nearly two decades of continuous study of his movement. He has pushed to the limits of what is possible in the absence of proprioceptive feedback, and pushed further than other patients with similar but less severe problems. If he was compelled to start a journey which few have ever thought of, his courage has taken him further than neurologists and physiotherapists could possibly imagine.

12

Senses and Sensibilities

So far we have considered the effect on Ian of his illness only in the most immediate terms of the loss of touch and proprioception and the resultant difficulties in movement. But our sensations cannot be considered in such simple and crude terms. The various types of sensation have profound effects on our feelings and thoughts - on our so-called affective natures.

The primary sensations – vision, hearing, smell, taste[1] and the touch/muscular sense – alert us to changing conditions in ourselves and in our environment. Some alert us to events close to us, or in us, while others can respond to incidents at a distance. They prepare us for, and help us with, the guidance of movement: they alert us to danger. Through them we gain information about the world and ourselves. But these sensations do not play upon us impersonally. They alter our emotional or affective qualities. Sherrington went as far as to say:

> Mind rarely, probably never, perceives any object with absolute indifference, that is without 'feeling'. All are linked closely to emotion.[2]

If we define the intellect as that faculty of mind by which it receives and comprehends, and the affective faculty as that by which it feels, the different types of sensations clearly have different access to, and influence on, these two aspects of mind. Since the intellect occupies the more accessible level of consciousness and is more able to have its contents communicated than our deeper affective natures, senses impinging more on the intellect may take a disproportionate amount of our consideration.

Vision has evolved to alert us to events happening some distance away and occasionally to guide our movements in relation to an object. (Rarely is it involved in guiding movements on its own, except during learning. Ian constantly has to use vision in that way.) Vision is also the sense that tends to dominate our thoughts and our intellectual faculty. Hearing may be placed a little way behind, while the other senses impinge much less on our intellects and less often on our conscious attention.

The influence of the senses on our emotional, more human natures, however, shows significant differences from their influence on our intellectual selves. Diderot considered the matter and concluded:

> I found that of the senses the eye is the most superficial, the ear the most arrogant, smell the most voluptuous, taste the most superficial and fickle, and touch the most profound and philosophical.[3]

The purpose of this chapter is to consider whether or not Diderot's claim is correct: to consider how the illness robbed Ian not only of touch but of those affective qualities which arise in us from sensations of touch and movement, and to compare the 'feeling' qualities of the various primary sensations.

*

Smell and its intimate associated sense, taste, are not well developed in man. Though some connoisseurs of the malt might disagree, the sense of smell has few analytical overtones. But it is well represented in the affective side of our nature. Smells are almost always described in affective terms such as 'pleasant', 'delicious', 'repulsive'. Taste and smell also have the ability to release memories as they are perceived, as in Proust's famous madeleine cake sequence. It is as though a disproportionate part of memory (which is rarely purely intellectual but always coloured by our feelings) concerns smell. This is sometimes explained as being because the areas of the brain concerned in memory and smell are close together in the temporal lobes; people with epilepsy of this part of the brain often experience hallucinations of smell and powerful *déjà vu* phenomena. This may reflect the importance of these two in earlier evolution, in choosing food and differentiating family, friend and foe. Babies for instance soon learn to recognise the smell of their mothers. We can only speculate.

Vision appears to be less important as an affective sensation: likes and dislikes are far more prominent in smells than they are in sights. It is easier to observe than to smell something impassively. Visual images do of course move us, but they are usually representative or figurative: for example, a child crying or a view of beautiful countryside. Images which leave the figurative and become abstract may appeal more to our intellectual than to our affective sensibility. Abstract images can indeed sometimes worry us. Seeing a non-figurative piece of art we may exclaim, 'But what is it?', requiring a visual image to conform to experience and unable to approach it for what it is, in abstract. We may admire the idea of a late Mondrian but are less likely to be moved by it. It was the genius of the post-Impressionists to imbue their work with their affective emotions. Van Gogh's intensity of feeling is observed independently of whether the painting is of sunflowers, a field or a chair. In this century some art may have refined the intellectual idea to the detriment of its affective force.

Hearing may be said to occupy a middle ground. It can act in a purely instinctive protective way – loud sounds make us jump. But, especially in man, the ear has become the receptive organ of communication through speech, which in turn may communicate at all levels of our intellectual and emotional faculties.

In their turn words can be either spoken or written. Care should be taken not to equate the two. The spoken word contains more than just the words spoken. We gain information not only from what the words express but from the intonations, pauses, emphases and so on that a person uses. Thus a child learns to interpret her parents' voices before she learns language, and a dog 'understands' its master. Oliver Sacks describes a group of patients who had lost their ability to comprehend the words but not the affective milieu in which they were spoken.[4] They could still understand the deceptions of a politician's speech. One patient had the opposite problem. She had lost the ability to understand the affective quality of speech and so had to pay extreme attention to every word and insist that all words be used precisely so that she could deduce meaning from them. She had lost the ability to be moved by speech, however. She too saw through the politician's speech, not because of its hollow emotional appeals but because of its improper and inconsistent use of words.

Robbed of the additional affective quality it can employ during speech, written language can become more intellectual and less emotional. We would all be capable of communicating the contents of a room, or what happened at a cricket match in terms of runs scored, wickets taken, etc. We could describe the physical characteristics of our friends in terms of height, hair colour and so on. But it takes far more eloquence to distil and describe the affective characteristics of people. Eloquence is defined, not solely in terms of the appropriate use of language, but of its appropriate use in an emotional context.

The primacy of vision as a sense in our intellectual faculty, and the greater facility with which language acts as a mouthpiece for the intellect than the affective side of our natures, are reflected in the way visual images are more easily expressed in language than are sensations acquired through hearing or smell. There are far more words to describe what we see than what we hear or smell or touch. As our intellectual sensibilities develop, and perhaps predominate, we must be careful to preserve the precious use of language to express these affective emotional qualities, as well as to use it to communicate the more mundane facts and figures.

If hearing can isolate this 'feeling tone', the emotional message underlying the words of a speech, as shown in Sacks's example, it also has a far greater capacity to inspire in us affective feelings through its abstract sounds. Music has the power to move us immeasurably. Its abstractions can inspire and release an emotional range beyond the power of words. The rich musical traditions of Western culture show the range of feeling that sound can elicit, for, though beyond words, it is not beyond shared expression. Some music may appeal particularly to our emotions, while some – say, a Webern piece – appeals to our intellect. But, as in all great art, great music must be able to reach and stimulate all levels.

Another way the intellect is seen to be a more accessible level of consciousness can be seen in what happens if these senses are removed. The consequences are not as simple or straightforward as we might imagine at first. We may be able to imagine, or confidently think we can imagine, what it is like to be blind. If we were to shut our eyes, we would find it difficult to move around, to find things, and so on. But we would also lose the ability to look at faces to see the nuances of emotion that they transmit. We would have to rely on voices and sounds to reveal feelings and then begin to forget all visual images.[5]

Deafness, however, may even be beyond a simple empathy. To be deaf deprives us of much of the 'feeling tone' in communication and isolates the person in a way that blindness does not. Helen Keller, deaf and blind since a baby, wrote:

> I am just as deaf as blind. The problems of deafness are deeper and more complex, if not more important, than those of blindness. Deafness is a much worse misfortune. For it means the loss of the most vital stimulus, the voice.[6]

We can become blind temporarily by closing our eyes, though this gives little real idea of the world of the blind. With a little more difficulty we can also reduce our hearing, though this may be a long way from the experience of deafness. But we can neither divorce ourselves from the sense of touch and proprioception, nor even imagine such a deprivation. To be deaf or blind is, obviously, a huge misfortune, but at least there are others with similar problems. Ian had lost sensation in isolation, and was isolated further by the inability of anyone around him to understand his loss.

*

How then do cutaneous and muscular sensations fit in with this ordering of the affective relations of primary sensations? What does the loss of these perceptions mean to Ian beyond the 'simple' loss of ability to feel touch and move unconsciously?

As discussed above, it is difficult to divorce these sensations and movement, but in a few situations the cutaneous sense alone is stimulated, usually with changes in temperature. A hot bath, or a sauna, or lying lizard-like in the sun are stimuli to the skin alone and are considered relaxing, pleasant and even, perhaps particularly, sensuous. Cold wind on the face is refreshing, a shower enjoyable, not only for the temperature effect but for the feeling of water hitting one. All these are perceived by us and described in affective, not intellectual, terms. Ian has these sensations intact, though they are divorced from touch. He still gains pleasure from warmth on the face, but is rarely able to relax enough to allow himself to enjoy such feelings fully.

It is far more usual for touch and the muscular senses to be activated synchronously. These senses have large access to our feeling natures (even though the muscular sense has been adequately defined only in the last two centuries and is still without a general level of intellectual awareness in the general population). They are deep within us – such an essential part of us that little thought is ever focused on them. Yet there can be little doubt about the importance of these senses to our affective lives.

Sculpture or wood carvings in museums show the potency of the cutaneous and muscular senses in affective perception. The sign seen most frequently as we tour a museum or a stately home is 'Do not touch.' School teachers and parents repeat this endlessly as they lead round their charges. The fact is that we can see perfectly well what objects look like. But we apparently feel the need both to look and to touch, to explore with our hands and fingers the textures and contours of objects. Perhaps children know this better than adults. One of the appeals of Henry Moore's sculpture may be that, despite its abstraction, it has a sensuous quality. Though received visually, Moore seems to appeal also to our tactile sensibility.

When she was taken round galleries Helen Keller was allowed a full tactile exploration of sculpture. This of course was her only way of knowing a piece and she derived great satisfaction from it. So much so that she wondered whether feeling sculpture was a better way of experiencing what the sculptor was trying to express than seeing it.

Ian's tactile facility was deadened, all but obliterated, by the neuropathy, as he is well aware. But it doesn't prevent him from trying. I was with him in a laboratory once where there was an old computer terminal. Its keys and screen, instead of being angular, were set in a console of graceful curves, like a relic from a Star-Trek set. It begged to be touched, and I watched as Ian saw it and ran his hands over it. Though he couldn't feel it, the desire to experience it in the tactile as well as the visual domain persisted. When asked about this he agreed that he wanted to do it for that reason, even though he received nothing back. Old habits die hard.

*

Yet the contributions of the tactile and muscular senses to our affective sensibility are not limited to the exploration of external objects. They are perhaps more apparent in one's relations with ourself:

> The exercise of the muscular frame is the source of some of our chief enjoyments. The beautiful condition of both body and mind shall result from muscular exertion and the alternations of activity and repose...This activity is followed by weariness, and although unattended with any describable pleasure or local sensation, there is diffused through every part of the frame after fatigue a feeling almost voluptuous.[7]

Not so long ago the idea of running for pleasure was incomprehensible to most people. How could such a painful pastime be enjoyable? It must be masochism. But in fact running was for athletes, and is now for many other people, an enormously enjoyable experience. There seems to have been an awakening recently of a sense of kinaesthetic-related pleasure. Exercise is fun, but also provides a profounder pleasure. It isn't just that our cardiovascular systems are toned up and the risks of heart disease reduced. It isn't explained simply by the fact that levels of endorphins (the neurotransmitters associated with pleasure) increase in the brain after exercise. The sensations of movement, whether from running or riding or walking, may of themselves be felt as pleasurable: but pleasurable in a way so profound that the intellect and its mouthpiece, language, as Bell said, find it difficult to express.

This pleasure is not confined to humans. No: no one who has watched lambs playing, or a young colt running around a field, can deny that he is watching the animal enjoy the same pleasure in movement that we do.

It may also be suggested that movement reaches this affective level of appreciation when observed in others, especially in those movements perceived as graceful. Dance, and even some spectator sports such as gymnastics, give pleasure to observers as well as to the participants.[8] Ballet may express many emotions that language cannot – else why dance? But one constant is the pleasure of dance itself. Ian can no more dance than fly.

The enjoyment of movement we perceive in young animals also communicates itself to us. To see lambs gambolling gives us pleasure.[9] One of the most graceful of animals is the deer. It is no coincidence, as we have noted, that Ian, who is well aware of the losses of kinaesthetic sensibility his neuropathy has produced, turns to the forest to retrieve something of what he has lost from these fluent animals.

It appears to be a characteristic of this 'kinaesthetic' pleasure that it depends on and increases with practice. The more we run the more we are 'in tune with our body' and the more we gain from it. The fitter we become the more we enjoy running. The pleasure of dance depends on disciplined practice, at least in its higher forms. No one enjoys doing something badly. Practice makes perfect. It is one of Ian's tragedies that he has to impose tremendous control on movement but gains no satisfaction from improvement. He can't enjoy a walk for its own sake, nor can he relax feeling pleasurably tired after exertion. Despite his enormous self-discipline in learning to walk and walking he gains none of the affective satisfaction in return.

*

Thus far kinaesthetic pleasure has been considered only in terms of exercise. However, in many parts of the world it has evolved more subtly. In eastern cultures slow accurate movements and postures are attained by an intellectual concentration upon kinaesthetic patterns which are usually considered automatic. In Yoga and Tai Chi this volitional focusing on exquisite movement leads also to a profound movement-related satisfaction.

Conventionally, we regard the body as the servant of the mind, and believe that exercise releases tension and improves our mood. Nervous, agitated people are thought to express this in fidgety unharmonious movements. Yoga – and, in the West, theory such as the Alexander technique – suggests that the relationship is more equal, and that grace and harmony of movement and a relaxed and yet correct poise will lead to greater emotional and intellectual satisfaction.

This interaction between the use of our bodies and emotional and even intellectual calmness and clarity suggests that perhaps even our personalities may be related to our movements and gait. Before dismissing such theories, we should consider military training.

One of the first things army recruits are taught is to stand properly to attention and at ease, though they may have been standing perfectly well for two decades. Then, though they have been walking around for years, they are taught to walk again the army way. During the war patients in military hospitals even had to *lie* at attention for doctors' ward rounds. Soldiers no longer march, or stand to attention, in battle. So why this immediate and unrelenting concentration on imposing new postures?

Could it be that a person's posture and movement is an important part of his individuality and personality?[10] In the armed forces both are replaced by a collective identity, as the individual's self-esteem is fused with the regiment's. This may be necessary, not only to produce a more efficient fighting unit, but to reduce the individual's perception of his responsibility for his actions. The alteration of a person's movement and posture during military training suggests that the relation between kinaesthesis and personality may not be unimportant.

Our 'feeling' sensibility is affected not only in posture and locomotion. There are other movements which may be important. When we sit in a restaurant we put our feet under the table, and there they stay, relatively immobile. By contrast, our hands are constantly active – moving, fiddling and playing with the cutlery. During a lecture we may fidget and doodle on the paper in front of us. The hands, as Phillips remarked, are rarely, if ever, still for more than a few seconds.[11] It is as though they too have a need for exercise. Sherrington thus described Cajal, the Spanish neuroanatomical genius:

> Cajal's rich voice compelled attention to whatever he said. Of dark complexion, his olive-skinned face lit by brilliant eyes. His hands as he sat and talked seemed to ask to be doing something.[12]

Likewise André Breton on his fellow surrealist André Masson:

> Masson, right at the beginning of his career, invented automatism. The hand of the painter becomes his true ally: it is no longer a hand that initiates the shapes of objects, but one enamoured of its own movement and that alone draws involuntary figures.[13]

That may be a slight exaggeration, allowable – even expected – from a French surrealist. Yet the meaning is clear. At times the hand can appear to delight in its own exercise.[14]

What occurs is that we may make a voluntary command to move which is then translated by the neural apparatus into the correct signals for movement. We see the hand move and, while we may or may not have attended to the voluntary command, we are never aware of the intervening neural apparatus. If we have not attended to the volitional part of movement, or if the movement was initiated at a more automatic level, the origin of movement may appear to be in the hand. The fingers may seem to be moving by themselves for themselves.

Deprived of meaningful sensory return from his hands, Ian has to concentrate on finger movements above all others and they remain the most difficult of all his repertoire of movements. When he is not looking at his hands and using voluntary effort on them, they are still. In contrast Helen Keller's hands were alive, moving, constantly reflecting her thoughts and moods. Ian's hands and arms have lost that ability. They are deaf and so mute – mute and so dumb.

*

Thus far movement and posture have been considered in terms of their internal influence on the individual. But they are of course powerful methods of communication also. This has been known for years. More recently there has been an upsurge of interest in 'non-verbal communication' and 'body language'.

In children the relation between mood and movement is often fairly direct. A happy, excited child rushes round with loose-limbed abandon. A concentrating child will be still, eyes wide open, and perhaps with a finger or thumb in the mouth. A sad child may or may not cry but will curl up or turn away from the world. As children grow up, they learn to conceal their feelings not only in their facial expression but in postural control. Our body language may be so potent a reflection of our feelings that we need to reduce its eloquence to avoid vulnerability. Correspondingly, we may sometimes want to show our feelings at one level but not express them at another. Then we may use gestures which, though they may have been learnt, are generally understood in our culture. We use them appropriately and often, usually, involuntarily. We need to assume different guises, to act, both to avoid communication and to enhance it in various circumstances.

Since his illness, Ian has lost all this unconscious body language and is no longer able to employ the myriad body postures and movements we use in communication and deception. Fortunately facial expression remains. Ian is aware of this lack and, as always, has evolved ways of circumventing it:

'Sure, I realise that, say, to incline towards someone when sitting is a sign of affection. Remember, I was all right until the age of 19, so I had learnt all this movement behaviour by then. Now I sometimes use it, but only when sitting down, which allows me to do it without fear of falling, and I always have to think about it. I have to decide consciously to use my hands to move with and emphasise my speech.'

He has remembered and relearnt a limited repertoire of non-verbal communication which he now uses consciously when appropriate. To sit and talk to him is to see the arms and hands lifted up and down in front of him elaborating and extending the points made. On closer inspection, however, we realise that though the points are emphasised with the hands the fingers remain relatively still.

Ian is always caught in a trap. Isn't thinking about movement the same as acting? And doesn't acting suggest artifice or untruthfulness? Ian has re-learnt movements to get round, and also to reveal his thoughts. He has regained some appearance of spontaneity and the abilities to communicate and conceal his actions and hence his thoughts by body language. His reacquisition of body langauge allows communication, but in turn depends on concealment – concealing the fact that these gestures, which we all make unconsciously, are in his case heart-felt but consciously made. Given the severity of his illness, however, his resumption of body movements in this context, as an embellishment expressing feeling rather than simply a method of locomotion, like so much of his recovery, is remarkable.

*

This body language is apparent not only in our movement and postures but also in our choices of position relative to other people. We will stand closer to someone we like talking to than to someone we don't. Different individuals seem to need different amounts of 'personal space': areas around them that they keep to themselves. Ian needs to keep at a distance from others to avoid being knocked and to predict the movements of others. He also needs more space to himself and his movements, because his 'body image' – his perception of his own somatic self – is perceived no longer through the usual cutaneous and muscular senses, but through vision, and his postural movements are also less accurate that normal.

This raises the question whether his spatial awareness has itself been altered by viewing it rather than by feeling it. In *D'Alembert's Dream* Diderot wrote:

'What really sets a limit to the space you feel you occupy?'
'My sight and touch.'
'Yes, by day, but at night, in the dark, or even by day when your mind is preoccupied?'[15]

More recently A.J. Ayer considered this problem. He concluded that while 'one's concept of space is partly derived from one's experience of movement...there is no good reason why someone unaware of the situation of his own body and also deprived of kinaesthetic sensations should not only perceive spatial relations between physical objects, but also distinguish different places in his visual field.'[16]

Ian agrees with Ayer. As far as he can tell (and such matters are difficult to measure), he has a normal perception of spatial relations with his eyes open. In the dark, however, he would have no such perception, since he would be unable to produce a purposeful movement to explore extra-personal space and he would have no feedback of any movement he might make.

His perceptions of spatial awareness and his motor programs were built up during his normal childhood development. He is quite clear that without this he couldn't have recovered. Someone who had suffered from a sensory neuropathy like Ian's from birth would probably be devastated, being unable not only to learn movement under visual feedback alone but also being unable to construct a normal perception of extrapersonal space, even given the possibility that the immature brain has a greater ability to adapt.[17] Since such a hypothetical illness, thankfully, has not occurred, the argument cannot be confirmed or refuted.

*

The neuropathy not only deprived Ian of light touch and joint position sense. At first it prevented movement, and then it imposed severe restrictions on his movement and thought. It also lead to the loss of many levels and contexts of affective perception. The very depth with which these levels are felt may contribute to the difficulties of articulating them, and must have contributed to his difficulties in explaining what had gone wrong. His sense of touch was replaced by a sense of isolation, not only in his loss of touch and proprioception, but also in an almost complete inability to communicate fully its effects.

If the loss of sensation lead to obscure perceptual problems, the associated loss of movement was an obvious inescapable result. With this loss of mobility came the immediate need for full-time nursing care and complete loss of independence, with all the resulting inconveniences.

Yet there was also a deep sense of the loss of movement itself. In his poem Ian equated the living death, not with loss of touch, but with the subsequent loss of movement. Similarly Felice's first reaction on seeing her son was that he was a vegetable, because he couldn't move. The ability to move is an important aspect of our affective nature. Pascal wrote:

Our nature lies in movement; complete calm is death.[18]

Diderot echoed this:

Man is born to act. His health depends on movement.[19]

At one level all Ian's strivings to recover and to rejoin society have been a return to the land of the moving and hence of the living.

Comparisons of different classes of phenomena, whether they are works of art or primary senses, can be valid only up to a point. Yet Diderot's suggestion that touch was the most profound and philosophical of the senses may well be true. He must have had rare gifts himself to reach such a conclusion.

13

The 29th of February

Ian had become a valued member of John's statistical team despite the problems imposed on him by his illness. All the time he was at work he had to plan carefully. For instance, if he knew it would be busy he would plan the whole day out in his mind beforehand. If he had a meeting, he would have to arrange for someone to help him carry his paperwork. If it was late, he wouldn't do any photocopying earlier, in case he felt too tired to be useful later. If the meeting was formal, he would have to wear decent shoes rather than his preferred trainers. He would even cancel a social event the day before to ensure that he wouldn't be too tired to cope. He had to pace himself during the day, every day.

They were all very accommodating at work, but they had little idea of the continuing effort for Ian. As the years went by he was gradually taken for granted. That was a backhanded compliment to his functional recovery, but nothing had become easier for him. He had at first shied away from telling people too much about his disability, but he began now to discuss his condition with his colleagues. He felt that he owed them some explanation for his occasional absences from the office. But perhaps he was motivated also by his growing awareness of the strain he was placing on himself.

He had worked hard to achieve and maintain his independence, and to create a working environment in which he was accepted as just another member of the team. But he found it was becoming harder and harder to preserve the façade. He found himself questioning his motivation more and more. Once he might have just got on with it, but now he was becoming more analytical, and the doubts accumulated. Was the constant mental effort to be mobile and keep the job ultimately worth it? Was the financial security it brought worth the mental pressure involved? It wasn't the actual work that concerned him. He could cope with that perfectly well, and it posed no problems. No, it was the reasoning behind what he was doing that he focused on. He was concerned about what he had become by driving himself so hard. He was thinking, not of the past, but of the future:

'I felt I was burning myself out mentally. At first my motivation had gone when Mavis died, and it took me a long time to regain my self-esteem and self-respect. Then I began to realise that perhaps I was asking too much of myself. I began to think about moving back a step and taking life at less of a pace. But I wasn't really doing much anyway. All my energies were devoted to a rigid regime of work and household chores, with an occasional day off for excursions to the forest, as energies permitted.'

*

For the first time Ian began to think he might miss out on life before he had had a chance to enjoy and experience it. After seeing Mavis's life snatched away from her, he worried that a similar fate awaited him. He wanted to take a few chances, and use his energies for himself and his own enjoyment.

The new flat nearer work was the ground floor of a pleasant detached house. He moved in and decorated the kitchen. Though it turned out well, home was no longer important to him. He paid someone to adapt the bathroom into a shower-room and though he did the papering and painting himself he just couldn't give himself to it. It was a job that needed doing, and that was it: no more no less.

He now spent a great deal of time just pleasing himself. After work he would go out to the forest. He became a familiar figure among the naturalists and would swop gossip and sightings with them all. But he remained at heart a loner. Eventually he began to find that he was enjoying his visits to the forest less and less. It wasn't long before he noticed that his new self-centred life was an effort.

A year or so after he moved into the new flat, he heard that Linda had moved into a house nearby. She had just moved out from her parents' home, deciding that the time was right to become independent. Her friendship with Ian had left her confused. She didn't know what she had done amiss or how she had read him so wrongly. The episode had shaken her confidence, and she too had taken time to recover. Then she had decided on a fresh start. Buying her own house was the first step.

Ian felt that their living so close might be a good omen. He began to regret his treatment of her and to be sad that he might have lost her.

When he telephoned her she was surprised at first and then frosty. He had expected as much. But she rang him back a few days later. She was frightened and upset. She had always been afraid of spiders, she said, and there was a big one on her living-room wall. Could he come around and deal with it? Typically, he thought she was joking, but she soon convinced him she wasn't and he went around. The spider was enormous, and he was delighted it didn't make a run for it. He didn't fancy a slapstick half-hour tripping around her lounge trying to catch the damn thing.

As they chatted over a cup of tea he told her about Mavis and why he had stopped seeing her without an explanation. Her understandable suspicion and distrust melted as he told his story. He told her that he hadn't particularly enjoyed his time on his own. He had wasted time, something he had learnt to abhor. Though they couldn't undo what had happened between them, as the evening progressed they began to feel that their relationship could now be honest. Over the next few months they became inseparable. This time she told her friends in the office.

One morning Linda rang Ian at home as he was setting off for work. After talking for a while they decided to give the office a miss. They drove to Exmoor and had afternoon tea in a tearoom. They felt mad driving all that way just for a cup of tea, but that's what they did.

During the journey they discussed what they wanted for themselves in the future. They realised that they were all too obviously in love and decided they would live together, first selling Ian's flat and then Linda's house. They would buy a bungalow, and see what developed.

Not that their love developed smoothly. Late one evening they were driving over the top of a hill near Portsmouth. There had been snow some days before, but except for a few patches by the roadside it had all disappeared, or so they thought. As Ian turned into a little country lane, he saw that the road was completely blocked. He braked, but they were on ice and slid straight into the bank of snow. They managed to push the doors open. Ian suggested that with a little push from the front they would probably be able to reverse out. Linda wasn't amused, for she knew who would be pushing. She was relieved when Ian told her that she couldn't possibly get out into the snow with her smart shoes. The relief didn't last, for Ian offered her his wellies from the back of the car. They tried reversing out, with Linda pushing, but it was no use. Ian suggested clearing the snow from around the wheels. He didn't carry a shovel and told Linda to use a fallow antler, assuring her it would be just as effective.

By now he was helpless with laughter as he watched her trudging round the car in outsize wellies clearing snow from the wheels with an antler. Her amusement level was decidedly lower, and she began to fear for his sanity when he insisted she throw some bird seed, which he always carried in the car, under the wheels for traction. Eventually they broke free. Ian tried to convince her that one day they would both look back on the incident and laugh, but Linda wasn't convinced. He decided, albeit too late, not to pursue the subject, and they went home in silence.

On another occasion he was reversing along one of the Forestry Commission tracks deep in the forest when he lost concentration and the rear offside wheel ended in a ditch. Linda had to walk more than a mile to a phone to arrange for a breakdown truck with a crane to lift them out. To add a final touch, he realised he had no money on him, and she had to pay the bill. She was far from amused. At least life with Ian was never dull, which made a big difference from work.

*

They both knew by now that they would marry, but Ian proved a little slow in asking, perhaps because he was still not free of the past. So when Linda was in London on a training course she arranged for Ian to receive a red rose with a message on it saying, 'Will You Marry Me?', on 29th February. Typically Ian had also sent her one to the hotel, but without any messages. They spoke that evening and talked it over, but he was reluctant to discuss dates. It turned out that he wasn't worried about being married: it was the thought of being the centre of attention on the day that terrified him. He would have been happy to marry much sooner if they could have done it quietly. But Linda wasn't keen on that. The idea of a white wedding with lots of guests and all the speeches, photographers and the like might have left him cold, but he knew she wouldn't settle for less.

She felt they needed to be more positive and wanted to name a day. He eventually ran out of excuses and they started to plan.

Their announcement coincided with the move from the house into a nearby bungalow. It was in a fairly bad state of repair, so once more Ian set about doing a place up, only this time with enthusiasm.

They also bought Hannah, a bounding Airedale, and tried to train her:

'She is a joy and gave us both enormous pleasure. In keeping with her breed, she has no recognisable brain but she is a never-ending source of fun. It's amazing but she has the good sense to keep away from my feet though she's probably the clumsiest and most uncoordinated animal you can imagine. We were made for each other.'

They finished the bungalow two days before the wedding. They had decided on a small intimate celebration with just a few friends and relations, but slowly it escalated, as weddings do. Come the day, they had invited more than ninety friends and relatives. Linda did all the arrangements and made her own wedding cake, as well as all the buns, cakes and sandwiches.

Ian was content to leave the details to her. By now he was reconciled to the day's events. His worries were about the physical problems. Would he cope with all the movements involved in weddings – the kissing and all the altar business?

They decided on a beautiful old church at Portchester. The vicar was sympathetic and arranged for them to sit on chairs rather than kneel and to have the blessing at their chairs rather than at the altar. Ian was most worried about dropping the ring or not being able to place it on Linda's finger. He had visions of the whole congregation on its hands and knees struggling to find it.

Then, on the day, he got to the church and realised that he had managed to forget both the money and the certificates. Fortunately the best man had enough cash on him and the vicar accepted their word that the banns had been read in their parish. Ian's last hope of remaining a free man were dashed by a best man with a deep wallet, and an understanding vicar.

*

Portchester Castle stands at the head of Portsmouth Harbour. It was originally a Roman fortress with walls 180 yards long. Henry V stayed there before Agincourt, since when it has been used as a store-house for provisions and prisoners-of-war. The flat area inside the walls is now grassed, with a football pitch in the north-east quadrant. Squeezed into the south-east corner is a beautiful low Romanesque church. Built originally in 1133, it has suffered periods of disuse but has been restored each time. In the nineteenth century it was occupied by French prisoners, and it was they who, in 1816, planted the yew tree which stands in the walled graveyard. The previous tree had probably been killed by peasants with their kitchen fires.

The wedding was on a Friday in autumn. It was clear and bright, the day perfect apart from the cold wind that blew off the sea and tempted one to seek shelter. All Ian's family were there, except for his brother in the Foreign Legion. Mavis's brother and his family sat on Ian's side in a pew half-way back.

The service had the required solemnity. The ring wasn't a problem. Ian held it out and Linda guided her finger into it. Then we all trooped out, with the ancient bells pealing out above us.

We lined up outside for photographs. In the stiff wind Ian had his problems, but kept a grin throughout. The confetti blew horizontal in the wind, and I feared for him when he had a face-full by mistake. He tensed up and looked round for something to hold onto, but that was all over quickly. They went over to the keep for the more formal photos, a walk of a good hundred yards in the wind as the centre of attention, which didn't please Ian, but he had to do as he was told and survived.

At their house a scrum soon developed. Ian kept out of the way until things cleared a bit. With so many people round he couldn't venture into the crowded main rooms, but held court to a few friends at the back until the toasts and speeches.

When people realised I was a doctor they all wanted to know about Ian's illness and the research I had done with him. They said how well Ian had done. But all they knew of his disability was what he had chosen to tell them. They were amazed when I tried to describe what he lived through each day.

We had a few speeches with the usual jokes and platitudes before

Ian made the big announcement: he had finished doing up the bungalow and they were going to sell up and move away from the area.

*

After the wedding, Ian and Linda had much to sort out. Linda wasn't to return to the office. Feeling thoroughly frustrated, she had decided to look for another job and had been offered one with an insurance firm in Kendal.

For Ian the decision was more complex. The effort of working a normal 9-5 job was enormous and left him little mental energy for the rest of living. In the dark days he had dedicated himself to working, proving to the world and to himself that he could do as well as anyone. But more recently he had been pulled two ways. They had so much to do together that he needed mental concentration out of work as well as in. Sometimes he had been short with her after work. They both knew that he wasn't really like that. Yet the consuming motivation in his recovery had been to show that he could hold down a job. He now wanted to continue proving that, even though he didn't really enjoy his work, but also to have a life outside.

He had been given the opportunity to move into a new sphere at work, but it would only have been putting off the inevitable. It was the environment that was strangling him. He was becoming more and more disheartened by many of the ridiculous management policies, and it was time for a radical change and review of his situation.

The alternatives were to go part-time or to leave work altogether, at least for a while. Yet both would involve a degree of perceived defeat. One retreat from the normal world might lead to others. He had struggled with these ideas before and done nothing. He sought advice. Would he be giving up if he left? Would it negate his previous achievement? Could he really reconcile himself to retiring on health grounds when his whole motivation had been to overcome, even to ignore, the demands and effects of his illness.

For those around him the situation was simple. He had spent nearly twenty years driving himself with little thought of the long-term cost. We were worried he would drive himself too hard and end up with a severe back problem, or worse. In someone less resolute leaving work would have been less worrying. We could only keep reminding him how severe the neuropathy was and how far he had come in his recovery. Of both he needed reassurance.

'At first I was reluctant to leave on health grounds, as that would be a sure sign of defeat. But the more I thought about it, and the more I discussed it, the more I could see it made good sense. I looked on it as the ending of a chapter where I had made my point and succeed in holding down a job and competing with my able-bodied colleagues on their terms.'

The next question was what they would do and where they would go. They were both keen on the hills and had decided to go west or north. Linda would support them for a while, and they would take stock and perhaps work at their long-term ambition to run a tea-room or small hotel. They had been to the Lake District and had both enjoyed the freedom of the fells and lakes. They knew they could settle there. The offer of a job in Kendal was too good an opportunity to miss for Linda. She decided to take the job and started soon afterwards, before Ian gave in his notice. After living together for a year, they were forced to split up as soon as they had married.

A new project was being lined up for Ian at work. But his enthusiasm was waning. John had always realised that Ian wasn't temperamentally suited to working in a large organisation and that one day he would need to become his own boss. He had also seen that the demands of the illness were beginning to take their toll. So when Ian decided to call it a day he was hardly surprised.

*

John was sorry: they could little afford the loss of someone of his experience and ability. Still, they arranged a good send-off – under the code name 'Operation Russ', after Russ Abbott, a look-alike. It was the biggest leaving extravaganza they had ever put on, a 20-30 minute show of 'Ian - This is Your Life' before more than a hundred, a mock show in more ways than one. Everyone they could drag in was press-ganged into the elaborate secret rehearsals. Linda was up in Kendal staying in a company flat, and had to help organise from there. The weekend before the show she pretended to leave on the Sunday night to go back north but instead went round to stay at her parents', in order to surprise him the next day.

That Monday lunchtime they lured Ian into the trap, saying that a Welfare Officer wanted to speak to him. Ian was never fooled that easily and immediately rang the Welfare Officer. It was just as well they had arranged with her to corroborate the story.

'I remember walking down the corridor towards the Welfare Office when out of the canteen jumped Father Christmas doing his HO-HO-HO-ing and asked me to join him in the canteen. I recognised John, but thought he was dressed up for a children's tea party and declined the offer, saying I had an appointment. He insisted I join him and held the canteen door open for me. At this point I saw all the people and guessed something was up. I couldn't believe all the time and trouble they had gone to. I was surprised and amazed. They stitched me up good and proper. It was a great send-off, albeit a few weeks early. I was amazed at how devious and secretive Linda had been. I really thought that she was in Kendal.'

*

The first thing he promised himself was some time off. With the small settlement from his medical retirement he could afford it. He moved up to the Lakes and drove around absorbing the space and peacefulness. Freed from the need to work and plan, he was much more relaxed. He even looked better. He had gained a new perspective and sense of ease with his achievements and with his present circumstances.

One way this showed itself was in his willingness to think about the past. It was only in the last year or so at work that he had been able to talk about Mavis. After six years, and with the fulfilment of marriage to Linda, he was now able to approach and explore his previous pain. At the time he had been devastated and embittered. He had managed to close that episode off from his life and slowly start again. But he hadn't come to terms with it. In fact it was only from a position of equal satisfaction and fulfilment that he had been able to look back at all.

Plans for the future began to occupy him. Several friends came up to see them. As he showed them round the Lake District, he was surprised to notice how little information for disabled people there was available. There was the minimum stuff but never enough detail. How many stairs were there? How steep were the ramps? How distant were the car-parks? There was a world of difference between a 'Suitable for Disabled' sign in a guide book and the information disabled people really need in order to predict whether a place will be enjoyable or a nightmare. So he decided to write an insider's guide-book for the disabled. This meant going to many of the places and checking them out thoroughly and testing the landscape just as he had once checked the floor in the office.

'One of my early experiences was to visit a local place of interest which all the local guides and publications had indicated as accessible to the disabled. I was disappointed to find that the car park was up a slope, that the ground floor was cobbled and that for good measure many of the cobbles were missing. There were steps on the ground floor but the first floor could only be reached by a ladder. Though disheartened by the lack of sensible information for the disabled I'm not surprised, and clearly there is a need for my project.'

Once, on a holiday in Devon, he and Mavis went to a hotel for the disabled and were appalled. There were ramps and wide doors, hoists and car parks. But it was all so spartan, as though the disabled should be grateful for whatever they get. There were none of the small touches of kindness that make a good hotel. Why, he asked himself, shouldn't these places be just like other hotels but with the disabled bits added on?

So another plan he is now forming is to act as a go-between for disabled groups, providing them with lists of suitable hotels in the Lakes, or even to act as a guide himself. But his long-term aim is to set up a guest-house. With Linda's cooking and his energy he is convinced they could make a go of it, given the number of disabled in the country. After all, the good places soon become known on the grapevine and are booked up years ahead. Ian and Linda just need a few years to settle down and find the right place – like any other couple.

Ian's sense of humour hasn't been dimmed by marriage. One morning, Linda told me, he woke up and told her a dream. Linda, it should be remarked, is a wonderful cook but is not without a slight weight problem. Nor is a friend of hers, Joan, who gave a reading at their wedding. Ian had dreamt that he had won £6 million, which he had to spend fairly quickly.

'What did you buy, Ian?' Linda asked.

'I bought a house for my mother and one for your parents.'

'Yes, Ian and...'

'I bought my brother out of the Foreign Legion and set him and my other brothers up.'

'Yes.'

'And I have always wanted a Range Rover, so I went out and bought one of those.'

'Yes, and did anyone else get anything?'

'Oh yes, and I bought you and Joan a week in a health farm.'

At Odstock he had had time and the freedom to get back on his own two feet. He now has a similar freedom. But this time it gives him the opportunity to develop something from his dreams of the last twenty years. Against that, the discipline of work has gone and he has to motivate himself. With his disability this is no easy task. Still, he wasn't expected to walk again after the illness struck. Not only did he learn to walk, but he went on to do a job and be fully independent. He managed to leave the world of the disabled behind him. Now he wants to give back to that world something of what he has learnt on his journey. It won't be easy, but it would be rash to bet against him.

14

The Daily Marathon

Twenty years ago Ian was a young man with the prospect of a lifetime in the surroundings he loved in Jersey. The illness ended that at the age of 19. In the first years of his recovery, when he received in-patient care in Jersey and Southampton and rehabilitation in Odstock, and in the years since, he has experienced the limits of living without Bell's sixth sense. He has matured as a person and has had to learn about his illness. All those chronically disabled who can should become experts in their own condition. When the illness is almost unique it is even more important.

He has also had time to reflect on his care. Things appear differently to him now from how they appeared at the time.

'The neurologists at the Centre seemed in control, and busied themselves with tests, which at first helped restore my confidence. But they offered little comment on what was happening or what the prognosis might be. One afternoon I taught myself to sit up in bed unaided, and it was this simple act, though I didn't know it at the time, that was to become the key to all my rehabilitation. At this point I was sent home. To feel that someone somewhere had an understanding of the problems would have been comforting. Yet nowhere I turned could I gain any comfort. I was alone, and the more the doctors questioned the more I realised that they understood very little of my situation. I was devastated. All my optimism disappeared. I felt I was on the scrap heap, let down and deserted.'

It is difficult to look at his care retrospectively. The doctors hadn't seen anyone before with the same degree of loss. All their teaching and experience led them to believe that he would be wheel-chair-bound. A prime consideration may have been not to give him false hope. But it is difficult not to believe that if they had spent a little more time listening to him, talking to him, they would have gained a better understanding of his potential.

'At first it was good to be home, but I soon grew more and more concerned for the future. My mother wouldn't always be around. What then? Together we started a series of exercises. I was convinced that the people at the Centre didn't appreciate the consequences of my condition, and I began to form my own ideas about rehabilitation. But it was difficult to impart those feelings, and I felt very alone.'

At this stage Ian was in the same sort of position as a person who has just had a severe injury to the spinal cord, with little expectation of recovery, who goes through periods of depression, anger and despair. He had the additional burden of the rarity of his illness which was beyond the understanding of those around him. Once at home, he was isolated in a way the spinally injured are not. His discharge seemed to demonstrate both the doctors' impotence and, worse, their subsequent lack of interest. The next few months were the darkest of all: dark because he was angry at his fate, but also because his home situation was difficult and much of his anger was directed at his mother:

'The old saying is that you always hurt the one you love. I supposed that with her I could get away with it and that she would always be there for me. Looking back, I'm terribly ashamed of my abuse of a mother's love.'

The next event he describes was entry at the rehabilitation hospital:

'It was at this stage that I went to Odstock. I was rebellious, stubborn and arrogant in response to my frustrations about my disability. They had seen it all before. But I will always be grateful to the many staff I came in contact with, because it was there that I began to come to grips with my disability both mentally and physically. Though they appeared to understand the clinical loss, they never seemed to grasp its consequences. But they gave me the space to learn about myself and my disability, and for that I will be forever indebted to them.'

He sees his recovery as due to his own initiatives, helped to fruition by the staff, but not originating with them. It was difficult, at 19, to realise that the doctors, whom he had been taught to look up to and trust absolutely, didn't in fact know much about his illness. It took courage to decide that if he was going to improve he would have to follow his own way. At first he was concerned not to antagonise the physiotherapists. In practice he worked in parallel with them, doing their exercises but in his way and for his own ends.

'I began to realise that it was no use trying to regain mobility by conventional methods. I had to accept that from then on all movement would be governed by conscious thought. An irony at Odstock was that the more I achieved the more targets I set, as I refused to relinquish any ground gained. But there were times when I just switched off. Those around me often made me feel I had given up. Again, I was frustrated by their lack of understanding. These were breathing spaces in which I absorbed what I had learnt. Reluctantly I resigned myself to the fact that it was impossible to convey my situation to anyone else, no matter who. How can one explain a total loss of proprioception – a sense most people don't even know they have?'

He was well aware of Ted Cantrell's worry that he might become institutionalised. On the other hand he didn't think that the staff at Odstock were fully aware of how hard it was for him.

'Another pressure at that time was finding a way of earning a living. My total lack of enthusiasm for the subject annoyed people. But my sole aim was to become mobile. I wasn't sure I could apply myself to a job if all my concentration was geared towards being "safe". Even sitting at a desk required constant thought. But I knew I couldn't stay at Odstock, and when the opportunity arose to study in Coventry I went because it was the easier option. I was of course apprehensive, both about how I would cope in general and about the academic work. In Coventry I was among people who had mostly been disabled from birth or soon after. I learnt a lot from them. I was still uncomfortable with my own disability, and I went out safe in the knowledge that no one knew me. I was also able to explore some more personal relationships, which I hadn't done for some time. The course work was easy and provided a good springboard for a return to earning a living. On leaving Hereward College I took the plunge and obtained a clerical post, though I still had doubts about my ability to cope. Fortunately they were misplaced.'

*

In spite of all the hard work there can be no doubt about the enduring loss which he first faced nearly two decades ago and which he faces daily. It is easy to forget, after all the successes at Odstock and later, that the illness allows him no rest nor time to forget, that it imposes its limitations on his movement all the time he is awake and parts of each night too. What are his regrets?

'I wish I hadn't been so hard on those around during the difficult times I was trying to come to terms with the disability and with myself. I did at least have the satisfaction of knowing what I was going through, what it felt like. Those around me could only watch, wonder and worry. In my frustration I turned in upon myself and shut people out. It must have been hard for them to understand.'

His first regrets are about the effects it has had on others:

'I wish I hadn't been as hard on those people around me, especially my mother and later my wife. Mavis was also disabled, so she at least had sympathy with what I was going through, and I met her after the worst for me was over. But for my mother, and to some extent my brothers, on whom I really took out my anger and frustration in the early days, it must have been very difficult. To cope I have become selfish with my time and energy, and I analyse constantly the benefits of carrying out any task. This makes me somewhat misanthropic, though I try hard not to be. Before my disability I would have considered myself an optimist. Underneath I still am. It's just that to survive I have to tackle life very differently from how I would wish. I try to be as self-reliant as I can. Often this causes problems with friends and family and I feel I have been too quick to rebuff their offers of help. To accept it would probably have helped to build a bond particularly with my family, but probably I built a barrier instead. At times I think I tried too hard.'

Again the effect on others. Disability never affects one person in isolation. The disabled are not only handicapped by their difficulty in walking or hearing or whatever. Because of that difficulty they must concentrate more to circumvent it, and this need for selfishness in turn reduces their ability to do other things, isolating them yet further.

'I hate not being able to socialise as I would like and always having to be in control of my situation. I think I have learnt to disguise my frustration at not being able to join in as one of the lads. Nevertheless it still hurts not being able to let off steam and let myself go occasionally. I get annoyed with myself as I feel my limitations must impose restrictions on others, and on bad days it is difficult to cope with. I have often had to turn down an outing with friends at the last minute because of the inability to cope on that day. It is asking a lot of people to expect them to accept that.'

Ian thought long and hard about going out with Linda, not because he didn't want to, far from it, but because he knew that being with him would reduce her range of activities.

'I demand an awful lot of friends, as sometimes I have to cry off at the last moment, because I just can't face the effort of doing something. I don't often go for a drink, because the places are crowded, and I rarely go to the theatre or cinema, because of the dark. I've been told I get away with it, partly because of my personality and partly because allowances are made. But I do analyse things more, not just for me, but how others are able to cope with it. I tend not to go to places, so others don't have to be with me and restrict their own activities. I do have feelings I sometimes hold back. I feel awful sometimes asking for help, having to give in to my disability and accept that there are things I can't do. Most times I find a way round – it's my pride, my bloody pride.'

In retrospect some of his personal regrets are for things he didn't do:

'I regret not having travelled more. Thinking sensibly I went to work first and planned to relax and gain enjoyment later, not realising that later my chance would have gone. But I mustn't dwell on that – you can get very negative, and I've been down that path. You're on a hiding to nothing.'

Despite that he remains toughest on himself, both in what he has achieved and in the continuing effort involved:

'I'm no hero. I just get on with my life and make the best of it I can. I get good days when I can cope with the pressures of daily living and bad days when all I want to do is run away and hide. That's very hard to get across to some people who see you everyday and try to encourage you, and naturally want you to do your best. It's difficult to get across to them that today, unlike yesterday, you just can't handle it. I drive myself hard to compete and survive in a normal world, maybe too hard sometimes. But for me it's sink or swim. There's no middle ground. I feel that to live at a level lower than I know I'm capable of would be giving in.'

*

When I was in Oxford doing research, I had a colleague in the lab, Bill, who was a good enough rower to be one of the token Englishmen in the Blue Boat three times (winning each time) before being selected to row in the Olympics. He would spend three or four hours a day training, from autumn till Easter. Much of this was in anaerobic repetitions, beginning where the Jane Fonda 'burn' leaves off, pushing himself harder and harder, learning to ignore and control the pain of the exertion. 'No gain without pain,' the coaches would shout through their megaphones from the launches as the blue boat steamed up and down the river. Bill reckoned that lobotomies might help the crew to keep rowing and not think about the agony.

The limits to endurance in sport, whether in rowing, athletics or cycling, appear to be physical. Yet paradoxically the test is as much one of intellectual concentration. Pushing yourself day after day beyond what your body wants requires a severe mental discipline. The aim of training is as much to learn that mental concentration as to improve the performance of the muscles and heart. In this context the brain can indeed be viewed as another muscle. There is a cost though. Bill, my colleague, would return from an afternoon on the river physically exhausted. He would come back, collapse and wait to be revived with tea and buns.

But he was just as tired mentally and intellectually as he was physically. He made little progress in his research during his intensive training periods. Movements which are normally automatic had to come under a degree of voluntary control during training, not of course because the motor programs had broken down, but to impose from above the command to keep going in the face of painful signals from the muscles that they had had enough.

If in normal subjects mental concentration upon movement is tiring, it is even more tiring in those with neurological problems. Alf Brodal, the neuroanatomist, who had a stroke leaving him with a weak left side, wrote:

It was a striking and repeatedly made observation that the force needed to make a severely paretic (weak) muscle contract is considerable. Subjectively this is experienced as a kind of mental force, a power of will. In the case of a muscle just capable of being actively moved the mental effort needed was very great.

This force of innervation is obviously some kind of mental energy which cannot be quantified or defined more closely. The expenditure of this mental energy is very exhausting, a fact of some importance in physiotherapeutic treatments. To a lesser extent it is felt in all innervations of paretic muscles when they get tired, for example in walking when one has to concentrate on the process of moving the leg properly, in contrast to that for a normal leg.[1]

Brodal, who had experience of both normal and abnormal tiredness, implies that the degree of tiredness is far worse after neurological damage. Yvonne Moir describes how disabled children can advance in their school work or in physiotherapy, but cannot concentrate on both at the same time.

In one of the examples given above conscious effort was used to move a limb made weak by a stroke, and in the other it was used to move a tired and pain-producing muscle. But in both cases this effort was intellectually tiring. Ian has to use this same mental effort, not because he is weak, but because he has no way of using automatic programs. All his movements require intense concentration. He has to be at his best simply to get by:

'It may sound arrogant, but I have to live at my peak. I'm always at my maximum ability. Some athletes may do it in runs and races, but then they only have to reach a peak once or twice a year. I have to be there every day and without the reward of glory or prestige that may motivate an athlete. It takes so much effort to do anything, it's often all I can do to cope with it; but I have to keep on.'

In fact nearly all disabled persons have to live at their peak just to get by each day. If they are not at their peak they have to make a decision to live at a lower level of functioning at which they are comfortable.

Another time he was feeling low and said in a rare moment of candour:

'I'm trying not to sound melodramatic and I'm sorry if it does, but sometimes I wake up in the morning and the knowledge of how much mental effort I'll have to put in to get by makes me feel down. It's like having to do a marathon everyday, a daily marathon.'

This marathon is performed on his own, without training partners or fellow athletes: a secret marathon known to and understood by him alone.[2]

He couldn't really understand this, let alone express it to anyone, during his period of rehabilitation, but the problems he was wrestling with did manifest themselves. During his stay at Odstock he occasionally failed to appear on a Monday after a weekend at home with his mother. This was sometimes taken as youthful rebellion. In fact it was because he couldn't face the exhausting schedule at the hospital. After he had left Odstock his mother remembers how tired he became sometimes:

'Often he'd start a job and be too tired to finish. For instance, he would volunteer to wash the car but after doing two wheels would say he couldn't do any more and ask me to do it instead. He'd go inside and make some tea. I'd be washing away for an hour and still no tea. He'd just fallen asleep. I found him like that several times, once in the garden trying to build a brick wall.'

Sherrington's saying that mind concerns itself with ends, not means, in movement, to allow itself time for other thoughts, is relevant.[3] Ian cannot think of much else when moving. Automaticity in movement frees us from the mental effort of constantly directing movement. Ian has discovered how much effort it entails.

One would imagine that every so often he would decide to have a rest.

'Yes, I have to say 'Stop'. I've got occasionally to do nothing. Before I had family commitments there was a time when I lived alone, and then Christmas Days were quite good. I used to see no one, just do my own things. I'd come back afterwards just the same, but I'd have had a rest. I'd give myself breathing space and not force myself to do certain tasks. I'd reduce the pressure, not to have to think.'

Despite his physical problem, he values these short breaks in terms of not having to think. If it is difficult to imagine his neurological lesion, with no touch and no perception of posture and movement, it is even more difficult to imagine the mental effort involved in directing that movement for the whole of one's waking life.

The problems and pressures of constantly 'living at your best' may partly explain why some disabled (and able-bodied) people adopt a level of functioning below their capacity. Performing at 'peak' day in day out requires effort and implies a lack of reserve if anything goes wrong. Others around you may also feel the disappointment if you can manage something one day and not the next day. Ian has no alternative but to live at his peak. Otherwise he couldn't function

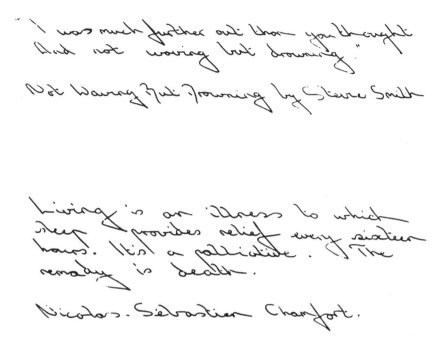

Figure 9. Examples of Ian's recent handwriting. 'My writing today is not good. It is slow to construct and lacks fluidity of style. I also have another style which is totally illegible to others, and sometimes to myself, which I use when I need to write quickly and take notes.' The first quotation from Stevie Smith appeals to Ian, the second he chose out of sardonic amusement.

usefully at all.

Ian's lack of reserve is seen most when he has a cold. The first time he had a cold after the illness all the gains of the previous months evaporated and he ended up almost back where he was, able to sit in a chair or lie down but do little else. He just couldn't cope with feeling rotten with the cold and the effort involved. He was really worried that his repertoire of re-learnt movements might never come back. But slowly it did. Even today he can't keep going while suffering from a cold and has to take a few days off. During severe colds he may end up in bed simply because he can't think well enough to be up and about. He carries with him the knowledge of just how vulnerable he is to the effects of such commonplace infections.

Just as his mental concentration for movement is limited in focus or field, so it is limited in time. He is aware of the need to conserve this 'effort' every day. He knows there will be few rest days for the remainder of his life. If he decides to do one thing, it may mean that he can't face doing another:

'I choose things I know I will enjoy, because it's so difficult and tiring for me to do anything. I don't want to waste effort. It makes me less adventurous, but at least I know I'll survive.'

After he started work in the statistics office he was called to an employment review and asked if it would help if he did some physical exercise or physiotherapy. He could only reply that, if he did, he would have little mental effort left over for work and daily living.

Occasionally he does do some simple gym work, under supervision. He determines its duration and extent, with an eye on what else is happening that day. Not only does the physical effort tire him mentally, but he appears particularly sensitive to the feeling of 'jelly' in the muscles after work, and this can interfere significantly with his walking afterwards. He hasn't been able to do enough physical work to notice any difference in his walking or general fitness. It just became another movement task draining his mental energy, but one without any use, and he stopped.

He still has the problem of trying to explain to others, even doctors, what is wrong. On moving house he changed his GP. One day he went to him with backache and tiredness. The doctor immediately diagnosed depression and told him to pull himself together and stop exaggerating the problem. (This unfortunately is the usual reaction and the reason why Ian dreads having to go to anyone new.)

Having been down as few have, Ian knew he wasn't depressed. But he did end up nevertheless wondering if he was perhaps making too much of his problem. He was almost reassured to have some simple clinical tests at the hospital which confirmed the severity of his loss of sensation. But the doctor's reaction cannot be entirely blamed. The neuropathy is all but unique and extremely difficult, even for a doctor, to understand. Few, if any, who have met Ian and seen him walking round can quite believe the severity of his case.

Recently we went to London to perform some neurophysiological research. When we arrived we were met by the doctor, Geoff, with whom I was to do the tests. He asked if I had brought the patient with me just as Ian was getting out of the car. As I introduced them and I could see the doctor's professional inscrutability taking over: he appeared not to register surprise. Later he told me:

'I was apprehensive about meeting Ian for the first time. I often find it difficult talking to disabled people, as it can be hard to know how they feel about their disabilities. In addition Ian's, as explained to me, were unusual and difficult to comprehend. But Ian put me at ease as soon as I met him! He held out his big hand in a handshake of welcome before walking up the steps to my office. It was obvious that he didn't walk normally, but it was amazing he could walk at all. The time was a learning experience for me, not so much about the expected disabilities as about the unexpected strategies for coping with them. He always looked round before starting to walk, and I discovered that he needed to be sure that there was no one close enough to bump into him.'

Ian said afterwards that at lunch while Geoff was talking to me he was also observing Ian. It was only when we did the experiments, which in passing established the severity of the neuropathy, that he realised how profound Ian's loss of sensation was. But it wasn't simply the extent of Ian's recovery that surprised him. He told me:

'Ian showed such a good understanding of our interest in the way he had learned to cope. In addition he has a remarkable sense of humour, which was demonstrated best of all when telling us how we should be doing our tests, or that we had forgotten to switch on some vital piece of equipment.'

In fact Ian has always been quick to understand and help with the experiments we have dreamt up in the last few years. We have never done a test *on* Ian, but always *with* him.

While Ian has become reconciled to his doctors' imperfect understanding of his disease and hence of his problems, he has always been indignant at the poor understanding of the problems of disability shown by some Health Care professionals he has met. A Disability Resettlement Officer, for instance, who failed to place one person in employment in eighteen months, the social worker who came to him when he first returned home, the people who site disabled loos with such poor access. It soon becomes apparent talking to him that much of the problem is that they don't listen to disabled people and don't approach situations from their perspective. Now that he plans to concern himself more with such issues, he may be able to achieve some change.

*

Ian's chances of sympathy or understanding are lessened further by his cheerfulness. Even at the beginning, when he had lost nearly everything, he kept his sense of humour. His levity has even led some to question the seriousness of his illness. His mother has overheard people say, 'There can't be too much wrong with Ian. He's always so cheerful.'

Someone at the office once thought him casual and flippant, though of course his work showed he wasn't. In common with many who are in control of their work, he does not feel that serious matters must always be performed with seriousness. On the other hand he has to impose such a discipline on himself that, on his own admission, he tends to employ humour as a safety-valve and a smokescreen, to hide his mental concentration.

Another reason for his light-hearted manner is suggested by his past problems. After being struck down by such an illness and spending a year stationary, doubting if recovery was possible, he was brought face to face with depths of depression and anger that few of us ever experience. Whatever casual claims he makes that 'anyone could have done it' he and only he knows the full effort and triumph of his subsequent recovery. After such an ordeal most of life's daily events must be viewed with less gravity.

In the epilogue to *Awakenings*, Oliver Sacks quotes Nietzsche:

Only great pain compels us to descend to our ultimate depths...I doubt if such pain makes us 'better', but I know it makes us more profound. One returns with merrier senses, with a second innocence in joy more childlike and yet a hundred times subtler than...before.[4]

He adds:

There are some hells known only to neurological patients. Those who return are forever marked by the experience. The effect is to make them not only deep but childlike, innocent and gay...they survived not as cripples, but as figures made great by their endurance, for being...undaunted and finally laughing...maintaining an inexplicable affirmation of life.

Ian may agree with all this but publicly he just shrugs it all off, saying, 'life's no bloody rehearsal'. He has had his bitter period and seen what it has done to him and those around him. Not liking it, he has slowly pulled out of it as best he could. There is no doubting, however, that he has returned from his own unique neurological hell changed in a way similar to that described by Sacks.

Part of that special hell is realising that to cope with the illness one's personality changes, perhaps leading to a selfishness and a shortness with others which add to the impoverishment of chronic illness. Ian is well aware of this:

'I often ask myself what it has cost me to survive with my disability and what sort of person I have become. I know what I am, and know what its done to me.'

Those around him can only assure him that he has overcome it. He returned not merely to exist but to enhance his life and the lives of others. The send-off he received at work was ample testimony to that.

In the right circumstances, and reading the mood of the person involved, it is often better to share laughter with the afflicted and disabled, thereby emphasising a common humanity, than to proffer sympathy which can underline differences. To quote Christopher Nolan:

Look, he begged, look deep down; feel, he begged, sense life's limitations; cry, he begged, cry the tears of cruel frustration; but above all he begged laughter, laugh, he pleaded, for lovely laughter vanquishes raw wounded pride.[5]

Laughing with someone implies an equality between you which tends to dissolve the frontiers between the normal and the disabled. Understanding this instinctively, Ian invites us to share not his sadness but his laughter. To mistake this for frivolity is like admiring the grace of a ballerina or the speed of an athlete while seeking to deny the foundation of their skills in discipline, effort and training.

'Humour played an important part in my recovery. An ability to laugh at myself and many of the situations I got into became so important. Though people couldn't understand my condition, at least we could communicate through humour. Humour relieves the tension of some difficult situations. It can be a shield to hide behind. Though this may be seen as a way of not facing up to a situation, I prefer to see it as a way of coping.'

Even this understates the case. Everyday humour may be ephemeral; by its nature it is hard to record. But it is the sign of a willingness to share one's life and open up to others. To retain this quality after an illness such as Ian's, and to be remembered in an office because of it, shows an extraordinary generosity and richness of spirit. Humour is not simply a shield, since it welcomes rather than keeps out those around: it is an invitation to share.[6] As Richard Feynman said, 'the highest forms of understanding we can achieve are laughter and human compassion'.[7]

*

Ted Cantrell has seen many difficult cases in rehabilitation: patients who started promisingly but then 'burnt out', who turned their backs on the chance of further recovery and settled into a less demanding role. Ian's neurological problem was, and is, so complex that such a pattern was expected. Indeed the plateau of a wheelchair existence was tacitly admitted both by Ted Cantrell and Yvonne Moir. Yet after his initial period of mourning Ian took his disability on, and succeeded against, and beyond, the expectations of the qualified observers.

Batsmen have been dropped by Test teams not because they failed to score runs but because they scored slowly and unimaginatively. In some aspects of life it is not enough to do the task: it is also necessary to do it with enthusiasm and enjoyment. If this is particularly true of sport and the performing arts, it is also true of everyday life in general. The characters we all like are those who obviously enjoy what they do, the larger-than-life characters, the life-enhancers.

That Ian should return to a normal job and live independently was more than all the professionals expected. But he did far more than return to normal life; he returned with relish. At work he was popular because he was encouraging to those around him. His spirit hadn't been dragged down by the illness but had soared above its miseries. Linda once said that it was his humour and joy of life that first endeared him to her, before she knew he had anything wrong with him. He is a tight-rope walker who does impressions at the same time.

After his illness, for the first three years of his slow functional recovery[8] he had to concentrate on himself, squeezing advances from endless repetition and thought. Lesser men might have given up. How did he keep going? 'He was arrogant, bloody-minded, selfish, awkward and stubborn.' That was just the opinion of his mother. He himself puts it down to pride. But his self-esteem is tinged with doubt:

'On a bad day I despise myself for having created such a monster, particularly when I acknowledge that the prime motivators in my recovery and determination have been pride and vanity. Yet on a good day, if I push myself to the limit to experience a spectacular view or take a difficult photograph, I am elated by a sense of achievement. At times like that I allow myself smug and conceited thoughts.'

He wasn't going to let it beat him and he was going to 'prove the buggers wrong'. His pride came before a fall. It came before many falls. Without his pride he wouldn't have stood up in order to fall. Without his pride he wouldn't have refused the catheter, or the wheelchair, or the ankle braces, or the special arrangements for exams. Without his bloody pride he might not have returned single-mindedly to the life of an able-bodied person, against the advice of many experts and the expectations of them all.

According to Ibsen 'the strongest man is he who stands alone', meaning a man alone with his principles.[9] Ian showed such solitary strengths at many levels and succeeded literally as well as metaphorically.

Pride may be defined as an inordinate sense of self-esteem. But we all need self-esteem to survive the vagaries and buffetings of everyday existence. In exceptional circumstances what is interpreted as pride may be all that's left, all that lies between a person and the abyss of going under. Without his self-esteem, his determination to keep it intact and his exceptional endurance, he would probably not have recovered. As Felice says, 'I could have killed him at the time, but he was right.'

While lying at home and in Odstock he set himself goals of returning to the real world and of living and working independently. Once he had achieved these goals, he found that the effort involved in sustaining them slowly drained him of the enthusiasm essential for functioning. It became harder and harder, in his words, 'to psyche himself up enough': to say, 'Yes, I do want breakfast. Yes, I do want a shave. Yes, I do want to go to work. And yes, I do want to keep on living.' Many people who live alone, and most people over 65, find the same thing. It must have been particularly hard for Ian who for the most part was doing it on his own while few people around had the faintest idea how hard it was.

Having done something once, he allowed himself little sense of achievement, as there was always so much more to do. Yet it was scarcely less difficult to do it the second time, or the hundredth. With no way of transferring a newly re-learnt movement from the conscious to the automatic he had to concentrate on each movement each time. We may praise a child the first time she rides a bicycle or swims, but after that the skill becomes just that: a skill, unconscious, characteristic of the person yet not of their thoughts. Our individuality depends both on our unique ways of walking or writing – unconscious motor skills – and on the quality of our conscious thoughts and behaviour. They are almost indivisible in the eyes of those who meet us.

Skills become accepted and so forgotten: forgotten and so not worthy of praise. Ian wasn't looking for perpetual praise, but when he had managed anything once he had to maintain that same level of achievement to repeat it. A lack of awareness of the problem in others contributed to his sense of frustration and to difficulties in motivation. People's perceptions were based on normal subjects. The more Ian did the more he recovered, and so the more he could do and the less support he appeared to need. He became a victim of his own success. He could live with that, but at times he found it difficult to maintain his motivation.

Meeting Mavis rekindled his enthusiasm for challenges, his desire to enjoy and embrace life. Mavis taught him to get on with it, to be thankful and not bitter. The effort suddenly became worthwhile: it was shared. They took on challenging tasks, which neither could have contemplated alone. Together they learnt to savour and honour their precious lives together, never squandering or taking for granted levels of health which for many of us might be poor.

After Mavis died, the spark went out of Ian's life. What for many is a poetic or emotional truth was almost literally true for Ian. He returned to live an infinitely more mundane existence in a small set of rooms: a small life in a small flat. As he says now:

'I was lucky to find a wife who inspired and encouraged me. Much that I achieved was due to her inspiration and love of life. When she died I came close to giving in. I continued alone for some time, as much out of respect for her as from any plan or objective.'

Being alone, however, slowly dragged him down. At one stage he became more and more convinced that his days were numbered and that the flimsy 'normality' he held on to would come crashing in around him. That was why he decided to spend more time doing exactly what he wanted, trying to enjoy what life there was ahead in a way Mavis had been unable to.

There was still something missing, however:

'I was getting older and I knew I probably wouldn't be able to maintain my previous level of concentration. Naturally that concerned me, but it went deeper than that. I missed having someone to go home to, someone to talk to about personal and private things. I missed having someone to love and I missed being loved. Once again I felt I couldn't find enough justification to continue just for my own sake. I didn't like myself enough to feel that the effort was worthwhile. I needed someone to share my life with: someone who could make me feel that life was worth living, not just on the good days, but through the bad times as well.'

Now, after a period of some years, remarrying has given him the chance to begin to take life on once more. The change in Ian has been noticed by all. Jim and Brenda have noticed, even at a distance, how his sense of purpose and enjoyment was reawakened by Linda. He just says she lets him out of the washing up and the ironing. Indeed she does, but it might have been expected that with someone to share the daily chores Ian would have conserved what he has and done less. In fact, though he can avoid some of the tasks he finds difficult, his general level of activity has increased as he takes on new challenges. The balance between the sheer unrelenting mental tiredness of movement and the desire to enjoy life has been tilted gloriously by Linda. His old enthusiasm has returned and the awkward old bugger has resurfaced.

'Amazingly good fortune has come to me again, in my finding someone to share my life with. The effort of moving forward is worthwhile once more.'

*

Ian is obviously concerned for the future, since he doesn't know how long he will be able to maintain the mental energy required to keep going. In spite of all he has been through, in spite of all his achievements, and in spite of the happiness he now knows, the neuropathy remains. It is accepted but loathed:

'I detest being trapped in my body and not having independence and freedom of mobility without constant thought. I despair at not being as free as I was when younger, at not being able to walk the woods and fields as I pleased. I mourn the lost opportunities. Fortunately not all days are like these. I delight in the fact that I have travelled far and that the road still intrigues me.'

Of one thing he is certain: 'I have come too far and have too much to look forward to to give up.'

But he is still refining aspects of movement with a conscious deliberation not known even to students of dance. Recently he went on a holiday to Jersey and met some friends he hadn't met for years. One girl ran up to him exclaiming, 'But, Ian, you can bend your knees!' While amused that after six years this was all she could say, he was pleased that someone had recognised a new movement. Being able to bend the knees even a little he has found to be terribly important in walking.

Having clawed himself out of a wheelchair by pride and self-reliance, he found it difficult to sustain that enthusiasm alone. Even in someone as disciplined as Ian self-absorption and self-preservation, 'pride, bloody pride', could only take him so far so long. He spent months, years, re-learning movements, re-learning to function independently so as to work alongside able-bodied men. Once he had achieved that level of functioning it wasn't sustainable by self-esteem alone. To return to a full life of enjoyment and satisfaction others had to be admitted. Mavis, and now Linda, gave him the motivation to sustain himself at his peak through the daily marathon. If the problem was in maintaining motivation, its solution has proved to be through the enhancement of life and its enrichment with and for another, through what many call more simply love.

Felice once said: 'It's remarkable to sit here and see him now, working, married and enjoying life. I always had visions of how I'd be pushing him round in a wheelchair.'

Remarkable it is indeed.[10]

Notes

Prologue

1. These experiments are discussed briefly as footnotes in Chapters 3 and 11.

2. I wrote to all the six medical authors who have described similar syndromes. Of those who replied none had continued to follow up the subjects.

3. Sir Charles Bell, *The Hand: Its Mechanism and Endowments as Evincing Design* (1833).

Chapter 2. Gastric Flu

1. The drug has never been implicated in the development of acute sensory neuropathy.

2. He had lost the sensation of touch and of feedback from his body. Phillips (1985, see *Movements of the Hand,* Sherrington Lecture XVII, Liverpool University Press) wrote: 'If it can be assumed that acute withdrawal of feedback were practicable in man, all parts of the acts of reaching and grasping would become impossible immediately.' He was referring to hand movements. Ian seems to have suffered such a fate, but also to have lost all positional awareness, from hands, arms and body. This prevented control of even the simplest posture, let alone use of the hand.

3. In some neurological illnesses the control of the bladder is affected. Distention of the bladder by urine can cause damage to the bladder and to the kidneys themselves. A solution is to put a small tube or catheter into the bladder to allow free drainage of urine.

4. This exceptionally rare occurrence will be considered in further detail in the next chapter. A similar case has recently been reported from Italy. (Caramia, M., et al., *Electroenceph. and Clin. Neurophys.* 1985, **66**, S17). The patient had a transient rash two days before the illness, and was found to have elevated anti-rubella (German measles) antibody titres in the spinal fluid. In this case, however, deep (muscular) sensation was affected rather more than cutaneous touch sensation. Ian appeared to have lost both. A causal relationship between the neuropathy and glandular fever has not been proved. The cause of the diarrhoea was presumably a virus which was never isolated. Neuropathies have been described in association with viral diarrhoea, and the glandular fever may have been incidental.

5. Limbo – the edge of hell, abode of souls to whom the benefits of redemption could not be applied, through no fault of their own.

6. He was treated with a course of steroid injections to reduce the inflammation. The efficacy of this treatment was never established and it has become less common. He also had a course of penicillin intramuscularly which he remembers for the pain.

This was given some time after the neuropathy had established itself and so cannot be implicated in the cause of it.

Chapter 3. The Physiological Loss

1. It is possible to stimulate the peripheral nerves, with small electrical shocks, and record the brain potentials which result through electrodes attached to the scalp. In Ian we showed a complete absence of the usual early potentials which are conducted along the fast sensory fibres. Instead we were able to show slower potentials conducted along the small myelinated, or A-delta, fibres. The fast potentials usually take 20 milliseconds to reach the cortex after stimulation of a nerve at the wrist. Ian's first cortical response was after 84 milliseconds, four times slower. (Cole, J.D. and Katifi, H.A., Evoked potentials in a man with a complete large myelinated fibre sensory neuropathy below the neck, *Electroenceph. and Clin. Neurophysiol.* 1991, **80**, 103-107.)

2. Sir Charles Bell was a doctor who practised in Edinburgh and London. He was one of the founders of the Middlesex Hospital Medical School where a ward is named after him. An anatomist, physiologist and surgeon, his scientific discoveries were based on observation and thought as well as upon experimentation. In the days before anaesthesia experiments on animals were done while the animal was conscious, and without painkillers, and must have been repellent. (Surgeons operated on patients under not too dissimilar conditions.) Bell wrote in a letter: 'I should be writing a third paper on the nerves but I cannot proceed without making some experiments, which are so unpleasant to make that I defer them. You may think me silly, but I cannot perfectly convince myself that I am authorized in nature, or religion, to do these cruelties – for what? – for anything else than a little egotism or self-aggrandizement; and yet, what are my experiments in comparison with those which are daily done? and are daily done for nothing.' (Sir Gordon Gordon-Taylor and E.W. Walks, *Sir Charles Bell: His Life and Times*, 1958). Of his surgical skills his biographers comment: 'The particular period of his surgical activity before the advent of anaesthesia prevented one of his gentle humanity from equalling the exploits of surgical competitors who were cast in a tougher mould.'

Charles Bell gave not only the first description of the 'muscular sense', but also of the 'Philosophy and Anatomy of Expression'. In this, in addition to his medical interest, he showed superb skill and accomplishment as an artist. His great work, from which all my quotations come, is *The Hand: Its Mechanism and Vital Endowments as Evincing Design*, published in the Bridgewater Lecture Series in 1833, reprinted in 1979. It contains several examples of physiology much in advance of the time, as well as cataloguing evidence for the theory of evolution enunciated later by Darwin and Wallace.

3. Sir Charles Sherrington, OM FRS (1857-1952). Fellow of Gonville and Caius College, Cambridge, 1887; Lecturer in Physiology, St. Thomas's Hospital 1887; Fellow of the Royal Society, 1893; Holt Professor of Physiology, Liverpool, 1895; Waynflete Professor of Physiology, Oxford, 1913; President of the Royal Society, 1920-25; Nobel Laureate in Medicine and Physiology with Lord Adrian, 1932. The most eminent neurophysiologist of the late nineteenth and early twentieth century. Most of his work was reported in scientific journals but he did write several books, of which the most widely available is *The Integrative Action of the Nervous System* (1947). The quote is from The Muscular Sense, pp. 1003-1025, in Schafer's *Textbook of Physiology* (1900).

4. Professor Charles Phillips, FRS, who recently retired as Professor of Anatomy at Oxford. The quotation is from *Movements of the Hand*, 1985.

5. These matters are obviously very complex, and there may be no firm distinction between movements which are automatic and those of which we are conscious. At different times the same movement may be either, as Bell discussed in the quotation about walking on a narrow ledge.

6. Henry Head, *Studies in Neurology*, vol. 2, 1920.

7. For recent accounts of work on active touch and the physiological basis of tactile perception and fine movement see G. Gordon, *Active Touch: the Mechanism of Recognition of Objects by Manipulation: a multidisciplinary approach* (1978). Recent experimental work has increased knowledge of these physiological processes enormously. The extensive quotation from Bell's work is not meant to imply that little has occurred since, but rather to pay tribute to his achievement in an age long before electrical recording techniques were available.

8. In most neuropathies both sensory and motor nerve fibres are involved. In those purely sensory neuropathies all fibre types usually suffer some degree of insult, so that in addition to reductions in light touch and joint position sense, pain and temperature perceptions are also affected. Purely sensory neuropathies do occur (for review see P.K. Thomas, in Dyke, P.J., Thomas, P.K., Lambert, E.H. and Bunge, R., *Peripheral Neuropathy*, 1984). A few cases have been reported of a neuropathy in which the predominant damage is to the nerves subserving joint position sense, but these cases had some preservation of touch. (Sternam, A.B., Schaumberg, H.H. and Asbury, A.K., The acute sensory neuropathy syndrome: a distinct clinical entity, *Ann. Neurol.* 1980, **7**, 354-358).

A case similar to those of Schaumberg et al. has also been described most eloquently by Sacks as 'The disembodied lady' (Chapter 3 of *The Man who Mistook his Wife for a Hat*, 1985), but she too had preserved touch to some extent. Two cases like Ian's have been described recently: the young woman from Italy (see Chapter 2), and a woman in Canada (Forget, R. and Lamarre, Y. Rapid elbow flexion in the absence of proprioceptive and cutaneous feedback, *Human Neurobiol.* 1987, **6**, 27-37). Interestingly, in the Italian case all special tests were negative except that there was evidence that she had had a recent rubella infection. The conclusion was that the neuropathy probably arose from a faulty immune reaction between the cells acting against the infective organism and the myelinated sensory nerves. This is similar to the conclusion of Ian's doctors.

Several cases of sensory neuropathies involving all modalities of sensation have been well investigated from a physiological viewpoint, by Rothwell, J.C., Traub, M.M., Day, B.L., Obeso, J.A., Thomas, P.K. and Marsden, C.D., Manual motor performance in a deafferented man, *Brain* 1982, **105**, 515-542; Sanes, J.N., Mauritz, K.H., Dalaka, M.C. and Evarts, E.V., Motor control in humans with large-fibre sensory neuropathy, *Human Neurobiol.* 1985, **4**, 101-114; Forget and Lamarre, op. cit.

But in these papers it was the physiology that was considered. These cases were also seen sooner after the original illnesses. The conclusions made about residual functioning, which was minimal, though valid at the time, might have had to be revised if the patients involved had had intensive physiotherapy and if the experiments had then been repeated after months or years.

I met Ian fourteen years after his original illness. Only Sacks, who met Christina two months after her illness and studied her for about two years, has written about the longer-term effects of such a neuropathy and its consequences for rehabilitation.

9. Without sensation from the limb to tell us where it is, most movement becomes impossibly imprecise. Some rapid and precise movements are possible without this feedback but these require much practice first. Movement without feedback was studied by both Bell and Sherrington.

The experiment of cutting the sensory nerves from a limb but keeping the motor nerves intact was performed and the effects described by Sherrington with Mott in 1895 (Mott, F.W. and Sherrington, C.S., Experiments upon the influence of sensory nerves upon movement and nutation of the limbs, *Proc. Roy. Soc. Lond.* 1895, **57**, 481-488). It has inevitably been repeated under various conditions subsequently.

However, both Bell and Sherrington also considered this cutting of sensory nerves in the horse, which was at the time a widespread procedure of economic importance. With the metalling of roads, horses, which were still used for transport, often developed soreness on their hooves, with subsequent lameness. In order to prevent them from feeling the pain, but not of course by reducing the cause of the pain itself or the damage to the foot, the sensory nerves from the hooves were cut. Their anatomical arrangement allowed this to be done without affecting the motor nerves. This practice of 'foundering' was quite commonplace.

Sherrington reported that 'the horse which goes lame from tenderness of the hoof, trots normally after neurotomy has rendered the whole foot insensitive'. Bell, however, had taken this matter a little further some seventy years before, perhaps because he was more intimately acquainted with horses: 'the consequence of which operation is that the horse, instead of moving with timid steps, puts out its feet freely, and the lameness is cured. If, however, we were to receive the statement thus barely, the fact would militate against our conclusion that mechanical provision and sensibility go together, being equally necessary to the perfection of the instrument. It is obvious, however, that there is a certain defect; the horse has lost his natural protection, and must now be indebted to the care of his rider. It has not only lost the pain which should guard against over exertion, but the feeling of the ground, which is necessary to his being perfectly safe as a roadster.'

Chapter 4. Down

1. Oliver Sacks wrote an account of his own rehabilitation after he broke a tendon connecting his knee cap to the thigh muscle above the knee (*A Leg To Stand On*, 1984). His recovery was slowed by a loss of ability to use the leg even after the tendon had been repaired. He had temporarily lost central nervous system control of movement as a consequence of the peripheral injury. As control was returning, he found he could not drink. Even a couple of drinks would make him uncertain once more of the leg (Sacks, personal communication). These two examples suggest that while movement memories are being reconstructed the nerve cells involved are much more vulnerable to disturbance, whether the cause is toxic as a result of alcohol, or infective as a result of viruses.

2. A person's reaction to illness often goes through several stages. There is an initial disbelief and denial, which may be replaced by anger, perhaps expressing self-pity. Once the new state of ill-health is accepted there is a period of depression. This is usually temporary, with the person emerging to continue his life as best he can with a stoicism and enjoyment of his residual capabilities which is often salutary and humbling to those who are not disabled. A recent study from Uppsala has shown that persons who are spinally injured, paralysed from the neck down, value their quality of life as highly after their accident as before, once they have been rehabilitated; sedentary activities replace previous activities such as sport.

Chapter 5. Outward Bound

1. Brodal, A., Self observations and neuro-anatomical considerations after a stroke, *Brain* 1973, **96**, 675-694.

2. Quoted in Sherrington, *The Muscular Sense*, in Schafer, op. cit.

3. The problems of re-learning motor tasks were discussed in detail by the Russian neuropsychologist Nicholas Bernstein in *The Co-ordination and Regulation of Movements* (1967). The book contains some brilliant observations on the mechanism of motor acts.

4. 'The complete act in its perfect form demands the mobilisation in due sequence of a series of complex procedures: here the time relation...is of fundamental importance. A want of chronological exactitude will throw the whole movement into disorder: its "kinetic melody" has been destroyed.' Head (from chapter on 'Chaos' in *Aphasia and Kindred Disorders of Speech*, London, 1926.) Luria often used the term, eg in *The Man with a Shattered World*, and it was also used by Bechterew in the last century (Sacks, personal communication).

5. In *The Songlines*, 1987, Bruce Chatwin gave the etymology of 'melody' as from the Greek for limb, suggesting that the song came with the limb and so with movement. Luria's observation of the musical quality in movement could be viewed, according to this theory, as a rediscovery or a completion of the circle. Chatwin's book is a meditation and exploration of the importance of migrations in 'primitive' man's psyche and in the development of a harmonious relation with his environment. He was considering the movement of man and families over large distances. Ian's recovery is an example of the importance of movement at a personal level. (It should be observed that Chatwin's theory is not one that is generally accepted. The Greek word *melos* can mean either 'limb' or 'song' – in the first sense it is found only in the plural – but it seems to be a mere homonym. The poetic truth, however, no doubt remains.)

6. Some people have detected the rhythms of walking in writing, especially in poetry: 'The question occurs to me – and quite seriously – how many shoe soles, how many ox-hide soles, how many sandals Alighieri wore out in the course of his poetic work, wandering about on the goat paths of Italy. The *Inferno* and especially the *Purgatorio* glorify the human gait, the measure and rhythm, the foot and its shape. The step, linked to the breathing and saturated with thought: this Dante understands as the beginning of prosody.' Osip Mandlestam, *Conversation about Dante*, unpublished in full, but quoted by Brown in his introduction to Mandlestam, *The Noise of Time* (1988).

Chapter 6. Sent to Coventry

1. '...practice, when properly undertaken, does not consist in repeating the *means of solution* of a motor problem time after time, but in the *process of solving* this problem again and again by techniques which we changed and perfected from repetition...in many cases, "practice is a particular type of repetition without repetition".' Bernstein, op. cit., p. 134.

2. 'Ordinariness, the extraordinary aspiration of cripples! Because not to be attained, or at least not without effort, the commonplace and banal become invested with glamour.' David Wright, *Deafness* (1990), p. 109.

3. To investigate Ian's perception of whole-body movement and orientation we have arranged a visit to Professor Mittelstaedt's laboratory in Munich. There Ian will sit on a giant slowly-rotating turntable and, in the dark, indicate his direction of rotation.

4. Though new patterns of movement can be termed 'tricks', this word has too glib a connotation for what is an important facet of neurological rehabilitation. The creation and adoption of new procedures of movement by the disabled are the means by which they regain function. Many of the 'tricks' are difficult to analyse and may be idiosyncratic, but they should be studied so that they can be understood better and others can be helped.

Chapter 7. Skinning a Cat

1. Making love was not as it had been before, but it was surprisingly close. He had some difficulty with posture, and sensation was less. Yet to make love, he discovered, had much to do with a mutual heightening of emotion. Most of the pleasure during intercourse, and even at its climax, came not from peripheral stimulation but from within, and in this he was no different after the illness from before it.

2. Old people often become more idiosyncratic as they age, caricatures of their earlier selves. Some disabled people's eccentricities may also become more evident after their illness. It may follow from this that their individual needs vary more than amongst a group of able-bodied people.

3. Sir Charles Bell, op. cit., p. 199.

Chapter 8. Coming Alive Again

1. Dostoyevsky: 'Man is a fickle and disreputable creature and perhaps is interested in the process of attaining his goal rather than the goal itself.' *Notes from Underground*, Penguin, 1972.

2. 'She was a woman who had been given that beautiful voice of hers more or less to make up for the collection of awkward mistakes her body represented. 'Mario Vargas Llosa, *Aunt Julia and the Scriptwriter*, London, 1983.

3. Ian was denied movement without concentration and effort, while Mavis had difficulty in moving her affected limbs at all. By contrast spastics are often condemned to suffer uncontrolled movement. That many people shy from the paralysed and the spastic shows how deep is the relationship between movement, person and personality. The depth of this feeling should not excuse its essential inhumanity. The human condition embraces health and disease. To accept and understand only one of these states reduces us to being spectators at half a play.

Chapter 10. Life's Work

1. Slippery floors are a problem to many patients with poor balance, as well as to some old people. Ward floors in hospitals are often shiny, and are kept shiny by cleaners. Sometimes there is the opposite problem with carpets, which may make an area more homely but make pushing wheelchairs more difficult.

2. One of Ian's proudest boasts was that he never fell over at work. He found much of the more complimentary parts of this chapter embarrassing to read, and asked specifically that I should dissociate him from them. They derive entirely from his colleagues at work.

3. Ian is constantly amazed by the siting of disabled loos in London. Some are in the centres of squares surrounded by busy traffic and are almost impossible for anyone in a wheel-chair to reach; and they rarely have a parking space next to them.

4. Helen Keller, blind and deaf from the age of less than two, also found solace in

trees (Helen Keller, *The Story of My Life*, 1903). While Ian is compelled by the neuropathy to observe things at a distance, Helen Keller, without vision and hearing, had to be close, touching everything before she knew it existed. She describes the pleasure of playing in waves on a beach for the first time, and of exploring the bark of trees and climbing over them. David Craig, in a book about climbing (*Native Stones*, 1988), wrote: 'Even if you walk out into the wilderness there is still a layer of artifact between you and nature – the sole of your boot. But to climb is to be intimate with the very stuff of our habitat.'

For Helen Keller trees were individuals and friends, especially in the time between her illness and the arrival of her teacher, Anne Sullivan. For several years she was in a world that was completely dark and silent. Anne Sullivan taught her language by pressure in her hand and so enabled her intelligence to be released.

Chapter 11. The Physiology of Cheating

1. Buendia refused a game of checkers: 'He could never understand the sense of a contest in which the two adversaries have agreed upon the rules.' Gabriel Garcia Marquez, *One Hundred Years of Solitude* (1970).

2. Bell, 1833, op. cit., p. 112.

3. For a discussion of posture and its mechanisms see J. Purdon Martin, *The Basal Ganglia and Posture*, 1967. Purdon Martin studied post-encephalitic Parkinsonian patients at Highlands Hospital and dedicated the work to them. Though much of his book concerns the abnormalities he observed, the last two chapters consider postural adaptations to stance and movement in general. He also described briefly a man without touch and proprioception over much of his body because of an astonishingly circumscribed knife wound to the spinal cord. One cannot help but contrast the complexity of the subject with the clarity and simplicity of its exposition. Purdon Martin discusses the roles of vision, the inner-ear balance organ and proprioception in movement and posture in both man and animals. His conclusions are directly relevant to Ian's mechanisms of recovery.

4. Children are not light on their feet either. They bang down without cushioning the shock by landing on the ball and so sound like elephants going upstairs. It is some years after they learn to walk that they have the need for, and acquire, the more refined and quieter step of adults.

5. Burnett, M.E., Cole, J.D., McLellan, D.L. and Sedgwick, E.M., Gait analysis in a subject without proprioception below the neck, *J. Physiol.* 1989, **417**, 102P. Some time after the experimental session for this paper Ian told me that it was not necessary for him to undergo gait analysis. Because all his movements had to be under conscious control he had a good idea of everything he was doing already. (Throughout our experimental sessions Ian has always been one of the team since he soon picks up our ideas and offers suggestions to improve our experiments.)

6. Sherrington, *Integrative Action of the Nervous System* (1947). Teachers of the Alexander technique suggest that this relegation of the means of movement to the automatic is responsible for much of the bad posture, and hence backache, that bedevils our society. The means, as well as the end, should command our attention.

7. Barrett, G., Cole, J.D., Sedgwick, E.M. and Towell, A.D., Passive movement-related cortical potentials with and without feedback in man, *J. Physiol.* 1989, **414**, 10P. Barrett, G., Cole, J.D., Sedgwick, E.M. and Towell, A.D., Active and passive movement-related cortical potentials in a man with a large-fibre sensory neuropathy, *J. Physiol.* 1989, **414**, 11P. The observations we made from Ian's responses allowed us to interpret data from controls properly.

8. Torebjork, E., personal communication. Frukstorfer, H. Thermal sensibility changes during ischaemic nerve block, *Pain* 1984, **20**, 355-361.

9. For a discussion of the corollary discharge hypothesis of the perception of effort, see Phillips, op. cit., pp. 70-75 and McCloskey, D.I., Kinaesthetic sensibility, *Physiol. Rev.* 1978, **58**, 763-820. Experiments we have performed with Ian provide evidence that he has no ability to perceive corollary discharge, but may be able to use the sensation from receptors of intramuscular tension (Cole, J.D., Observations on the sense of effort in a man without large myelinated cutaneous and proprioceptive sensory fibres below the neck, *J. Physiol.* 1986, **382**, 80P.)

10. In a study of a man soon after he had suffered a less pure sensory neuropathy than Ian, it was suggested that the major problem for him in using his limbs was his inability to keep them still (Rothwell, J.N., et al., op.cit.). This and other studies have not followed their subjects for long after the illnesses and so have not observed any recovery. Ian's case has implications for the prognosis given to such people and the effort given to help them. Ian has almost certainly recovered better than others with similar neuropathies. The Canadian woman with a somewhat similar neuropathy was wheelchair bound two years after the onset of her illness (Forget, R. and Lamarre, Y., op. cit.)

11. Bernstein, op. cit., pp. 107-108.

Chapter 12. Senses and Sensibilities

1. Taste, beyond the simple modalities of sweet, sour, salt and acid, is perceived via the same sensory organ as smell, located in the air passages in the nose.

2. Sherrington, Chapter on 'Cutaneous Sensation', in Schafer, E.A., *Textbook of Physiology* (1900), p. 974.

3. Denis Diderot (1713-1784) French philosopher and man of letters and, with Voltaire and Rousseau one of the three major figures of the Enlightenment, is best known perhaps for his work on the *Encyclopédie*. His main interest was in the natural sciences, particularly physiology. In *Lettre sur les aveugles* (1749) he advocated that the blind should be retrained to read through touch, something suggested previously by the Italian Cardano (1501-1576). Diderot recognised that science had to advance through experiment, rather than through observation and deduction alone. He also realised that animals had to adapt to their environments in order to survive and that there may have been change between animals. 'Why should the long series of animals not be the developments of a single animal. The intermediary between man and the other animals is the monkey.' (*Éléments de physiologie*). In *D'Alembert's Dream* (1769) he described the delusion of feeling extremely small or large, elaborated by Lewis Carroll in the Alice books. The experience may occur in forms of epilepsy. These quotations are taken from John Hope Mason's *The Irresistible Diderot*, 1982, London.

4. Oliver Sacks, 'The President's Speech', in *The Man who Mistook his Wife for a Hat* (1985).

5. John Hull has recently described the experience of losing his sight as an adult. He showed that blindness is, in fact, a very different world from that the sighted might imagine (*Touching the Rock,* 1990).

6. Helen Keller, op. cit. There have been several books recently published that try to explain the experience of deafness. Three of them (Harlan Lane's *When the Mind Hears: A History of the Deaf* (1984), and *The Deaf Experience: Classics in Language and Education* (1984), and Nora Ellen Groce's *Everyone Here Spoke Sign Language: Hereditary Deafness on Martha's Vineyard* (1985), were reviewed by Sacks in the *New*

York Review of Books for 27 March 1986. In Britain a collection of literary pieces from the hard of hearing was published as *The Quiet Ear: Deafness in Literature* (1987). David Wright has published a personal account of deafness together with a history of the condition (*Deafness*, 1969, 1990). Oliver Sacks's interest in the subject was kindled by being asked to write that *NYRB* review and he has recently published a book on deafness and sign-language, *Seeing Voices* (1990).

7. Bell (1833) op. cit., pp. 205-206.

8. Dance characteristically involves movement to music. Bell went on to stress these relations: 'There is ... the closest connection between the enjoyments of the sense of hearing and the exercise of the muscular sense.' It should not be forgotten that, when music is seen being made, while it may accompany movement and even echo it in its absence, its very production depends on some of the most accurate, intricate and rapid movement patterns achieved by man. Musicians spend hours every day learning and practising their movement skills. The great players are those who, having developed these skills, can then impose on them an individual and affective component. To watch a violinist play a Bach partita is to see a triumph of the 'movement brain' as well as the musical brain. One wonders whether musicians gain a kinaesthetic as well as a musical aesthetic satisfaction.

9. Age and facility of movement are almost inversely related: young children are never still, pensioners sit on benches in the park. Perhaps the pleasure in movement does not decline with age, but sadly the ability to move often does. Someone who has been able to maintain a more youthful posture appears younger and more alert than someone who has not.

10. In *Resurrection* (Penguin 1966) Tolstoy describes how a man is recognised by his friend in the street after a gap of twenty years, not by his face, which has altered markedly, but by his walk.

11. Phillips (1985) op. cit.

12. Quoted in Ragnar Granit, *Charles Scott Sherrington: An Appraisal* (1966), p. 37.

13. Breton on Masson, *Surrealism* (1971).

14. Tolstoy wrote in *Resurrection* of a similar thing in the voice: 'If they talked it was only to satisfy the physical need to exercise the muscle of the throat and tongue.'

15. Diderot, *D'Alembert's Dream* (1769).

16. A.J. Ayer, *Philosophy in the Twentieth Century* (1982), p. 222.

17. Helen Keller had a good sense of the space immediately around her and of her local geographical space. For instance, she wandered alone through her garden.

18. Pascal, *Pensées*, 1662, Penguin 1966, p. 238.

19. Diderot, *Eléments de Physiologie* (published posthumously, 1875). Translation from Mason, op. cit., p. 261.

Chapter 14. The Daily Marathon

1. Brodal, op. cit.

2. The use of the term 'marathon' is not as inappropriate as it may sound. Ian listened recently to a radio programme by David Hemery on the mental techniques used by champion sportsmen. These were very similar to those he had devised for himself. He wished he had had the advantage of such coaching early in his disability.

3. Sherrington, *The Integrative Action of the Nervous System* (1947).

4. Sacks, *Awakenings*, 1982 edition.

5. Christopher Nolan, *Under the Eye of the Clock* (1987).

6. Ludwig Wittgenstein, 'Humour is not a mood, but a way of looking at the world', quoted from Ray Monk, *Ludwig Wittgenstein* (1990), p. 529.

7. Richard Feynman, *What Do You Care What Other People Think?* (1989).

8. In medicine patients are occasionally thought to be exaggerating their symptoms, or perhaps even making up a symptom which has no organic cause. The problem is then said to be 'functional'. Ian's recovery wasn't based on any physical improvement either, and so could be termed functional in the opposite sense: recovery with no organic alteration.

9. Henrik Ibsen, *An Enemy of the People* (Oxford edition, 1988).

10. It would be facile to suggest that all the research that has gone into this book has not changed Ian's attitude to his illness and to its effects. When he has spoken of becoming more analytical, this is partly because he was often asked questions he hadn't previously considered and asked to recall events he had previously preferred to forget. Likewise his friends and relations were not simply asked their recollections but why they thought Ian did something in a certain way and what exactly the matter was. It is my hope and belief that, by confronting some of the ghosts from years past, he has been able to lay them to rest, and that by understanding more about his neuropathy and its effects he is in a better position to live with his remaining abilities and to decide his priorities. I hope that by realising his achievement compared with others he will be able to live a little more easily with the monster of which he sometimes talks.

Bibliography

Ayer, A.J., *Philosophy in the Twentieth Century*, London, 1982.
Bell, Sir Charles, *The Hand: Its Mechanism and Vital Endowments as Evincing Design*, Bridgewater Lecture Series, 1833. [Reprinted by Pilgrims Press 1979.]
Bernstein, Nicholas, *The Co-ordination and Regulation of Movements*, Oxford, 1967.
Chatwin, Bruce, *The Songlines*, London, 1987.
Chekhov, Anton, *The Kiss and other stories*, Penguin edition, London, 1982.
Diderot, Denis, *Lettre sur les Aveugles*, 1749.
—— *D'Alembert's Dream*, 1830.
—— *Éléments de Physiologie*, 1875.
Dostoevsky, Fyodor, *Notes from Underground*, London, 1972.
Dyck, P.J., Thomas. P.K., Lambert, E.H. and Bunge, R., *Peripheral Neuropathy*, London, 1984.
Feynman, Richard, *What Do You Care What Other People Think?* London and New York, 1989.
Gordon, George, *Active Touch, The Mechanism of Recognition of Objects by Manipulation: A Multidisciplinary Approach*, Oxford, 1978.
Gordon-Taylor, G. and Walks, E.W., *Sir Charles Bell: His Life and Times*, London, 1958.
Granit, Ragnar, *Charles Scott Sherrington: An Appraisal*, London, 1966.
Head, Henry, *Studies in Neurology*, Oxford, 1920.
Hull, John, *Touching the Rock*, London, 1990.
Keller, Helen, *The Story of My Life*, New York and London, 1903.
Mandlestam, Osip, *The Noise of Time*, London, 1988.
Marquez, Gabriel Garcia, *One Hundred Years of Solitude*, London, 1970.
Mason, John Hope, *The Irresistible Diderot*, London, 1982.
Monk, Ray, *Ludwig Wittgenstein*, London, 1990.
Nolan, Christopher, *Under the Eye of the Clock*, London, 1987.
Pascal, *Pensées*, Penguin edition, London, 1966.
Phillips, Charles, *Movements of the Hand*, Sherrington Lectures, XVII Liverpool, 1985.
Purdon Martin, J., *The Basal Ganglia and Posture*, London, 1967.
Sacks, O.W., *Awakenings*, London, 1973, 1982.
—— *A Leg To Stand On*, London, 1984.
—— *The Man who Mistook His Wife for a Hat*, London, 1985.
—— *Seeing Voices*, London, 1989.
Schafer, E.A., *Textbook of Physiology*, Edinburgh and London, 1900.
Sherrington, C.S., *The Integrative Action of the Nervous System*, Yale, 1906, Cambridge, 1947.

191

Tolstoy, Leo, *Resurrection*, Penguin edition, London, 1966.
Vargas Llosa, Mario, *Aunt Julia and the Scriptwriter*, London, 1983.
Wright, Davis, *Deafness*, London, 1969.

Index